DETOX

WITHOUT THE DRAMA

Lose Weight, Boost Energy, Reduce Toxins & Feel Your Best!

MICHELLE STACEY

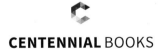

CENTENNIAL BOOKS

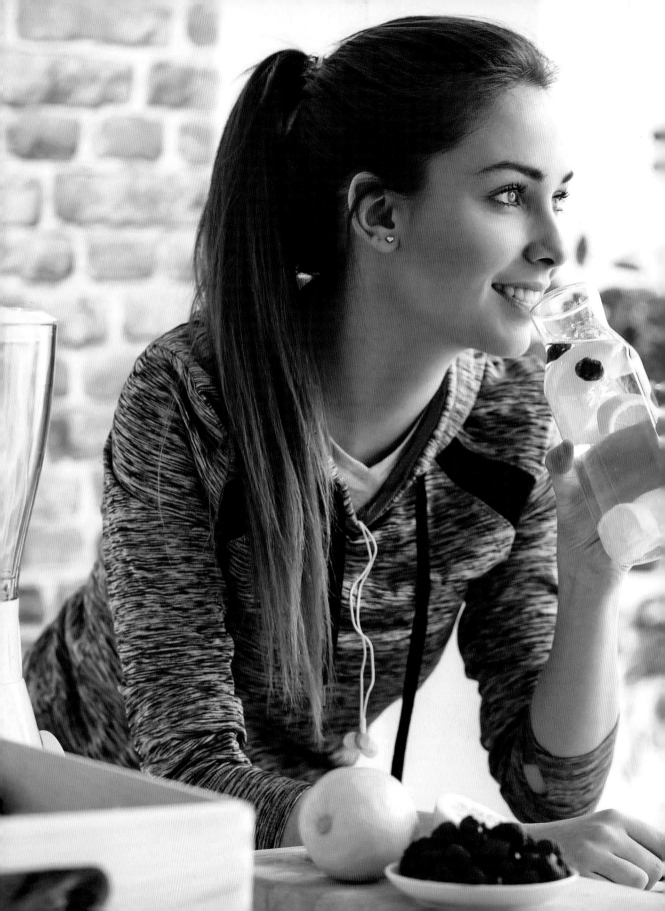

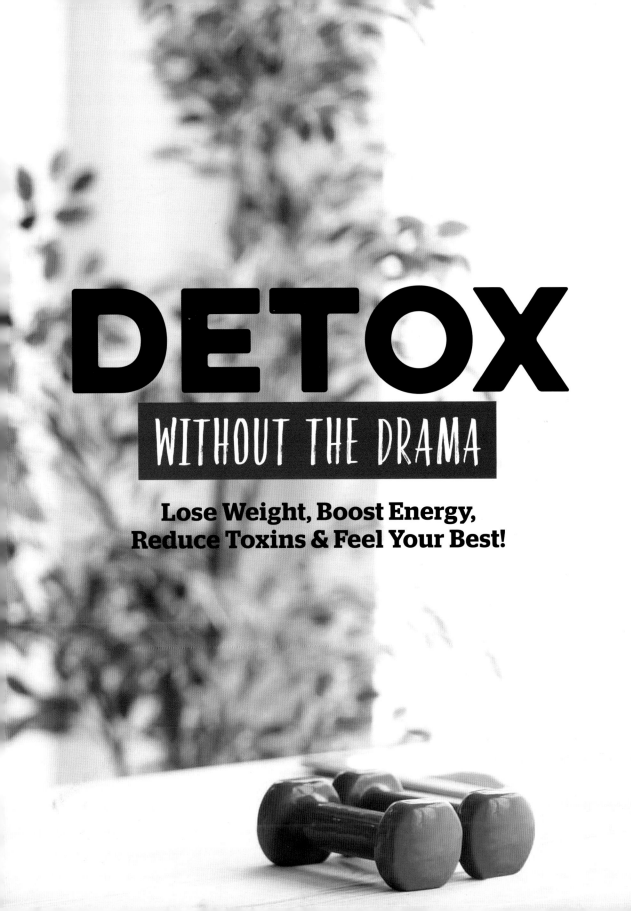

DETOX

WITHOUT THE DRAMA

**Lose Weight, Boost Energy,
Reduce Toxins & Feel Your Best!**

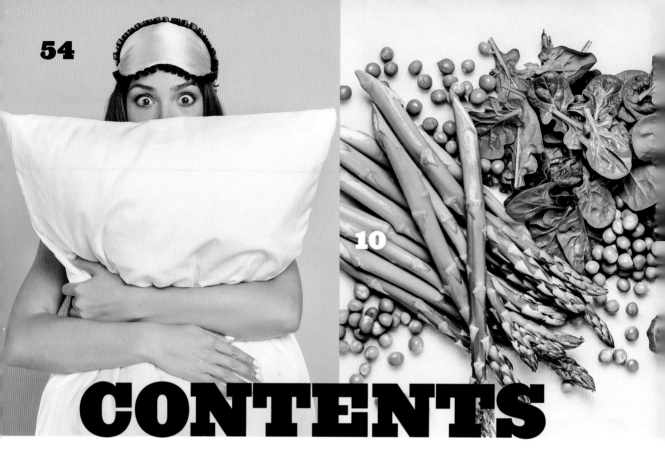

54

10

CONTENTS

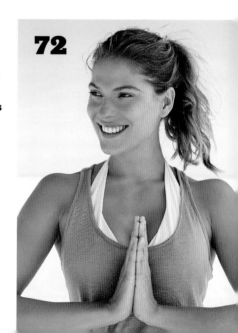

72

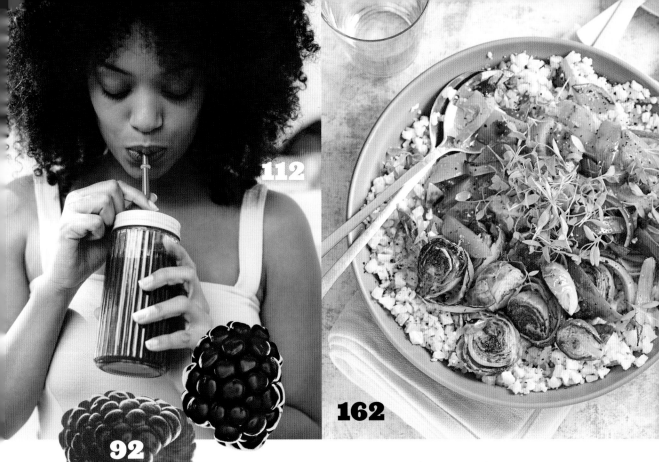

112

162

92

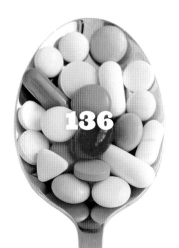

136

Get Back Your Bala

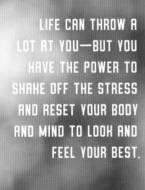

LIFE CAN THROW A LOT AT YOU—BUT YOU HAVE THE POWER TO SHAKE OFF THE STRESS AND RESET YOUR BODY AND MIND TO LOOK AND FEEL YOUR BEST.

Fnce

Feeling tired, sluggish, bloated? How about fuzzy-brained, hooked on coffee or riding a sugar-fueled roller coaster? Whether you blame modern life (it plays a part) or your own lack of willpower (go easy, now), you have plenty of company. These complaints are endemic, and lead us to an endless search for the perfect diet, exercise routine or lifestyle "prescription" that will cure all ills. But the human body is uniquely equipped to heal itself—to clear out toxins, repair cell damage, balance energy intake and more—if we give it half a chance.

The concept of detox does exactly that. Rather than a complicated protocol requiring expensive products and lengthy lists of "don'ts," the best form of detox involves getting out of your own way and enabling your body to use its own powerful systems of renewal. Detoxes and cleanses have sometimes been called reboots or resets for body and mind, and it's a useful metaphor.

Removing sources of toxins, unhealthy foods and behaviors unplugs you from physical and mental stresses and helps you return to your default settings, leading to a more healthful, even-keeled existence.

This book will give you a simple-to-follow road map to that reboot, walking you through what to discard (later, harmful chemicals and hidden sugars) and what to add (hello, good night's sleep, tasty food swaps, helpful supplements and an easy mindfulness practice). Need recipes for your reset? You'll also find delicious dishes that replenish your microbiome and retrain your palate (and cravings) for fresh, wholesome foods. Along the way you'll learn about the complex mechanisms that are doing the heavy lifting for you—the organs and systems that clean your blood, reduce inflammation and flush out harmful substances—and how they benefit from a detox.

The goal throughout is to harness the might of your own potent immune system—in a way that works for you, and without turning your life upside down. As you follow the steps laid out here, you'll find yourself feeling more energized, strong, clear-headed, calm—and likely, pounds lighter. In fact, rather than calling it a DE-tox, you could consider it a RE-juvenation: a return to a more youthful, more balanced self. Your body will thank you.

—Michelle Stacey

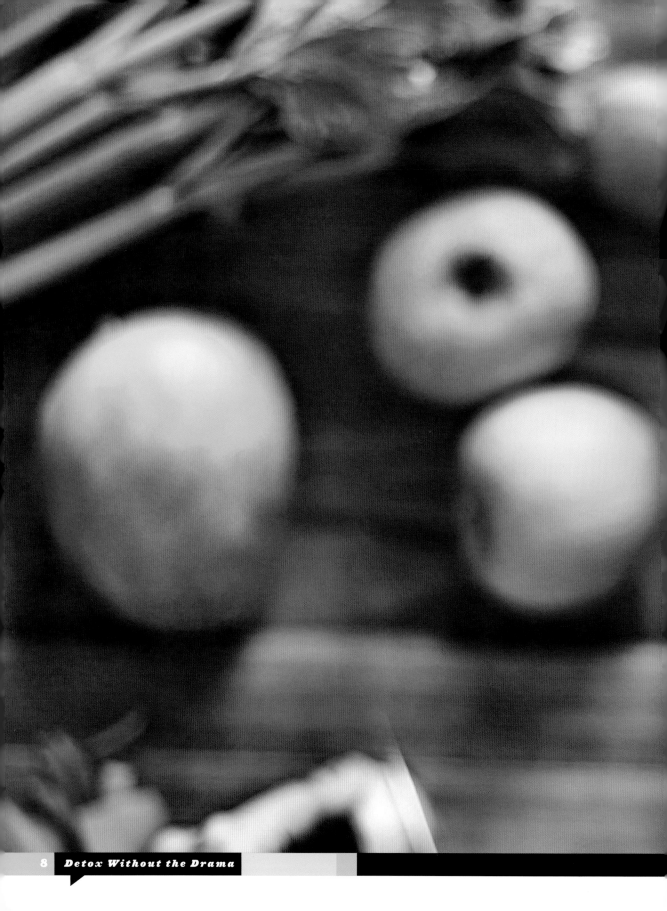

Detox Without the Drama

1

CLEANSING
101

EVERYTHING YOU NEED TO
KNOW ABOUT HOW DETOXING WORKS—
AND WHY YOU COULD BENEFIT.

A Clean New Deal

DETOXES AND CLEANSES HAVE A SLEW OF POTENTIAL HEALTH BENEFITS, FROM WEIGHT LOSS TO A STRONGER IMMUNE SYSTEM. WE SEPARATE THE MYTHS FROM THE REALITIES.

Greens are your new best friends.

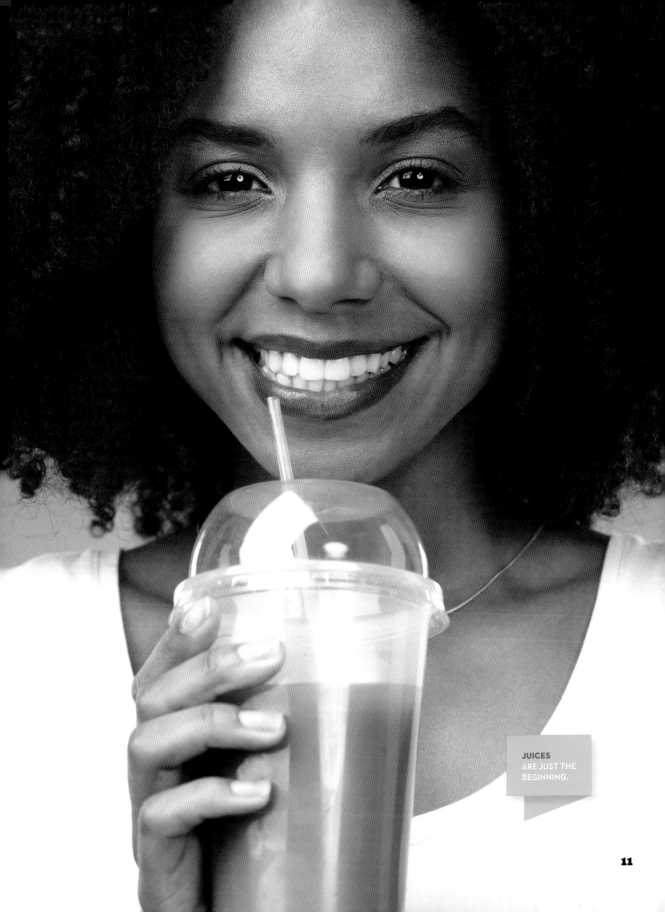

JUICES
ARE JUST THE
BEGINNING.

n common parlance, the verb "detox" once had a very specific definition—to quit an addiction to drugs or alcohol—and conjured up images of the Betty Ford Center. That began to change in a big way in the 1990s, largely spurred by the runaway success of the Master Cleanse (which itself was first introduced in the 1940s, but to a much more niche audience) and the rise of fresh-pressed juice emporiums such as Jamba Juice. "Dry January" has morphed into "vegan January," and Goop's annual January detox program takes it even further. In a similar way, old-fashioned detoxing from addictions has been broadened and redefined in the form of dozens of commercial mail-order cleanses, juicing benefits distilled into antioxidant-loaded juice "shots" (as in shot glasses) and detox programs aimed at specific body systems.

Though to many, programs called a "cleanse" or "detox" carry a whiff of new-age trendiness, the concept of periodically cleansing the body actually has a long history. "Body purification has been a part of mankind's rituals for health and well-being for thousands of years," says Linda Page, ND, PhD, a naturopathic doctor and author of *Healthy Healing*. "It's at the foundation of every healing philosophy."

Cleanses and detoxes have proponents and detractors, and misunderstandings and myths about these programs abound. If you're feeling that your system could use a healthy reboot, here's how to wade through the misinformation and separate the wheat from the chaff.

1 What's the difference between a detox and a cleanse?

"The terms are often used interchangeably," says Ansley Hill, RDN, LD, a registered dietitian in Portland, Oregon. "There's no 'official' definition or set of standards for a detox or cleanse protocol."

That said, there is a slight difference in emphasis between the two: "Detoxes tend to be more intense than cleanses, and operate on the notion that your body needs help eliminating harmful substances from your system," she adds. Cleanses focus more on cutting out unhealthy or allergenic foods—often sugar, processed foods, gluten, dairy and others—and replacing them with nutrient-dense whole foods. "Both types of diets are usually short-term and typically marketed for a specific reason, such as weight loss or alleviating general symptoms such as fatigue or brain fog," says Hill.

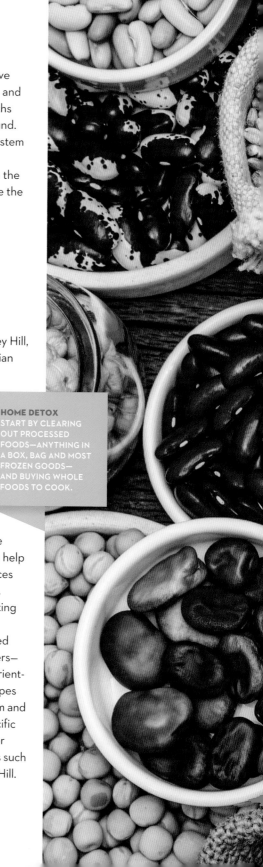

HOME DETOX
START BY CLEARING OUT PROCESSED FOODS—ANYTHING IN A BOX, BAG AND MOST FROZEN GOODS—AND BUYING WHOLE FOODS TO COOK.

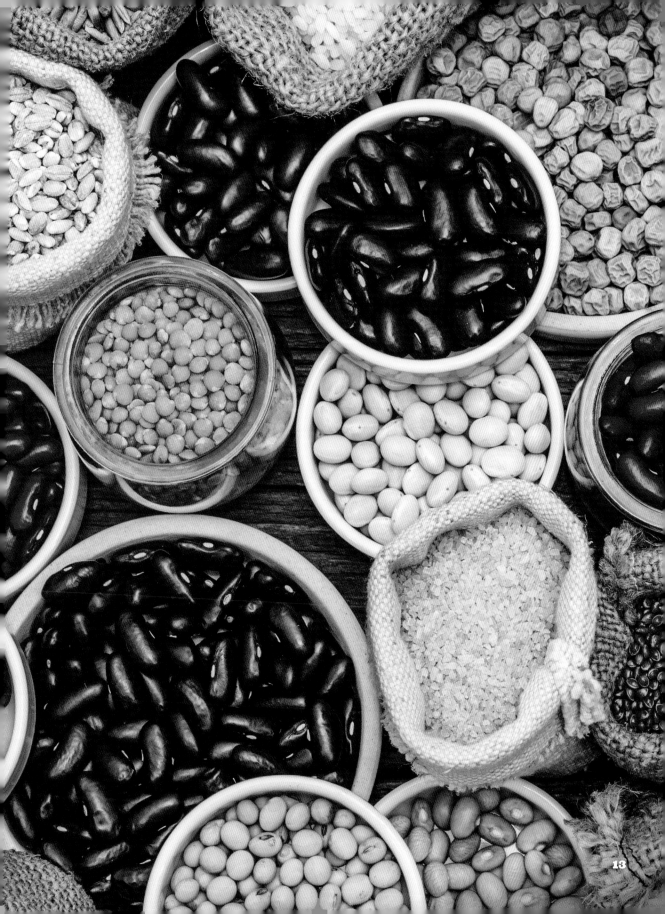

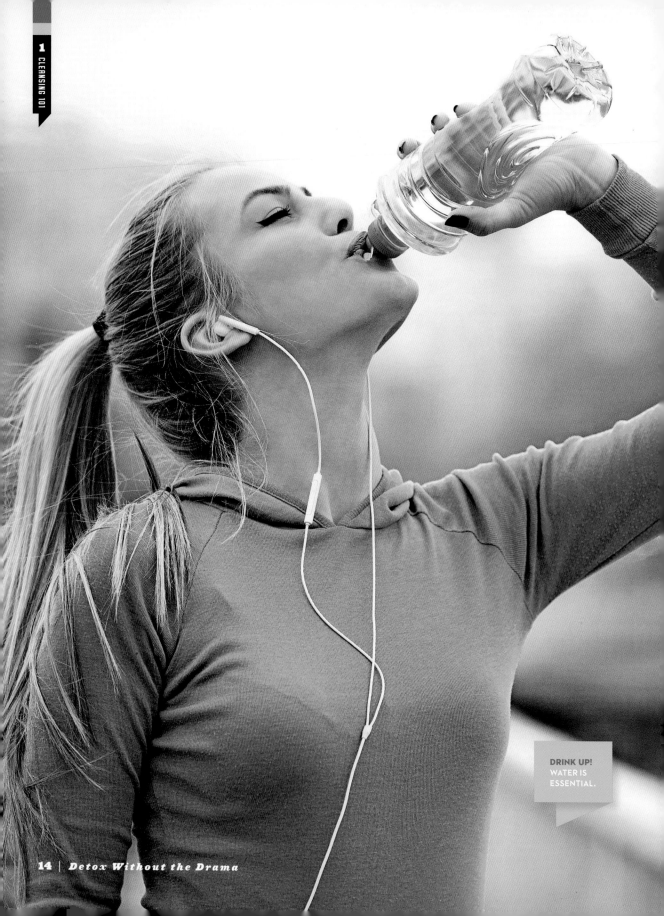

DRINK UP!
WATER IS
ESSENTIAL.

2 What are the potential benefits of a detox/cleanse?

There are many, says Page. First, a detox can "clear excess mucus and congestion from the body and clean your digestive tract of accumulated waste and fermenting bacteria." As a result, many people are able to turn around bad eating habits. "Detoxing can purify the liver, kidneys and blood in a way that's impossible under ordinary eating patterns, enhance mental clarity and strengthen the immune system," says Page. Lastly, she adds, if you feel you're dependent on sugar, caffeine, nicotine, alcohol or drugs, cleansing can help you break those habits. Detoxing gives your body a break from toxins and irritants found in foods and the environment that can harm health and cause weight gain.

3 Don't our bodies naturally "cleanse" themselves?

This is a point that many critics of cleanses and detox programs bring up, and the answer is yes—but that's not the whole answer, says Page. "Detoxification is the normal body process of eliminating or neutralizing toxins through the colon, liver, kidneys, lungs, lymph and skin." But there's

A detox can act as a *reset* to help nix bad habits.

a hitch, Page says: "Today, our bodies are fighting a losing battle. Systems and organs that were once capable of cleaning out toxic material are now overloaded, and much of it stays in our tissues."

Before the industrial revolution, people ate meals made from whole foods—not packaged goods pumped full of preservatives, produce grown with the help of pesticides, and livestock raised on hormones, antibiotics and other chemicals. They also breathed air untainted by fuel emissions, drank water free of factory waste and heavy metals and lived in structures without asbestos or lead.

"Our bodies are swimming in toxins," says Peter Bennett, ND, co-author of *7-Day Detox Miracle*. "We're constantly exposed to multiple toxins found in our medications, food, water and the air. Toxins that damage the cells of the body are invisible and insidious. They break down the 'invironment' of all body systems at the cellular level." That proliferation of toxic sources, Bennett says, "demands, more than ever, that we consider detoxifying our bodies."

4 Cleanses are expensive, right?

Not necessarily. If you choose one of the commercial cleanses, yes, it could be very costly. Many of these involve buying crates of bottled juices (sometimes supplemented by protein drinks), some of which can cost hundreds of dollars. But the other way to cleanse—and arguably the healthier way in terms of not only your bank account but also in the freshness and lack of processing in the foods and drinks you are consuming—is very inexpensive. It involves things you can easily

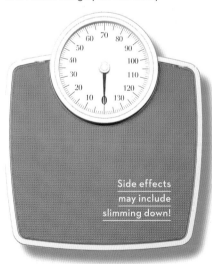

Side effects may include slimming down!

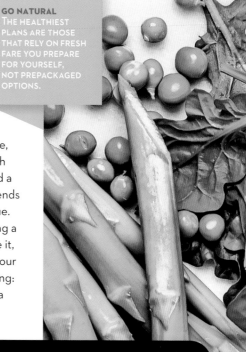

do at home and will likely result in spending even less money than you do now on groceries, including tea and whole foods that you prepare for yourself at home. You'll find the details throughout the rest of this book.

5 Is this all about weight loss?

Not at all. Weight loss tends to be the selling point for many cleanses, but the naturopathic doctors who are the greatest boosters for detoxes and cleanses place far more emphasis on the many health benefits that these processes can bring. That's

not to say you won't lose weight: Most people do, whatever form of cleansing they choose. That's because laying off processed foods, alcohol and other toxins and an unhealthy sedentary lifestyle, in favor of interventions such as exercise, better sleep and a diet of clean, whole foods tends to lead to a trimmer physique. But the other results of doing a cleanse, however you define it, may be more important to your health—and more far-reaching: greater vitality, energy and a longer life.

GO NATURAL THE HEALTHIEST PLANS ARE THOSE THAT RELY ON FRESH FARE YOU PREPARE FOR YOURSELF, NOT PREPACKAGED OPTIONS.

Cleanse Do's and Don'ts

Not all detox programs are created equal. Here's what to sign on for—and what to steer clear of.

RED FLAGS

- Removal or exclusion of an entire food group.

- Vilification of specific foods or ingredients.

- The notion that these specific protocols or products will vastly change your body chemistry.

- Specific promises of outcomes or results, aka "You'll lose X pounds in X days" or "You'll

rejuvenate your liver after completing these simple steps."

- Use of shaming or aggressive language, e.g., "Your food is poisoning you!"

- Requiring you to make a purchase (for instance, buying a certain supplement or series of juices).

- Use of a "one-size-fits-all" approach—offering one answer for everyone's health or digestive issues.

GREEN FLAGS

- A plan that can be done from your own kitchen, rather than commercially made products.

- Eliminating added sugars (many commercial juice cleanses, for instance, are high in sugar).

- A program that calls for using organic and local produce.

- Flexibility: You should be able to adapt your cleanse to

be gluten-free, vegan or inclusive of meat, for example.

- You should feel reasonably sated, not constantly hungry.

- It should include numerous sources of fiber—such as beans, fruits and vegetables—to help improve gut health.

- You should have enough energy to be physically active during the cleanse or detox.

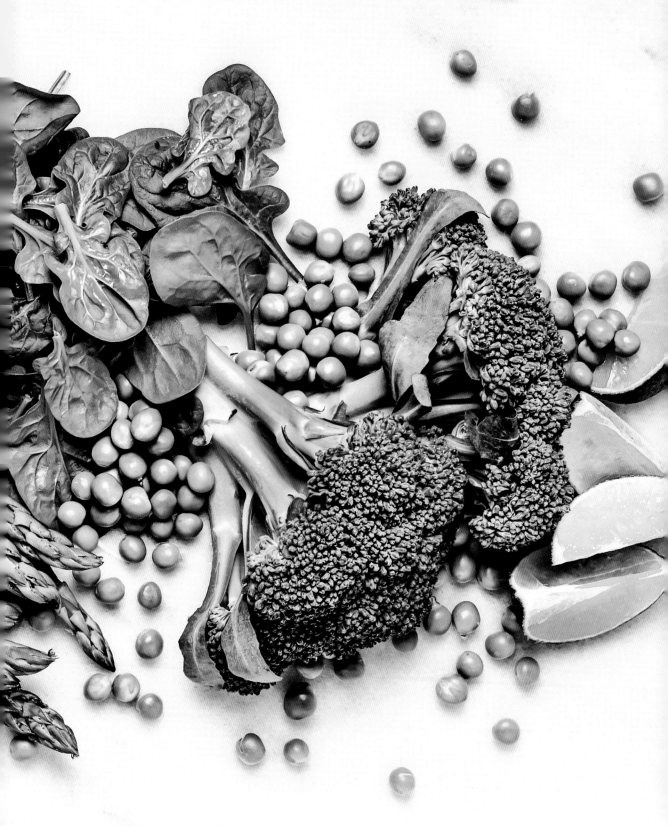

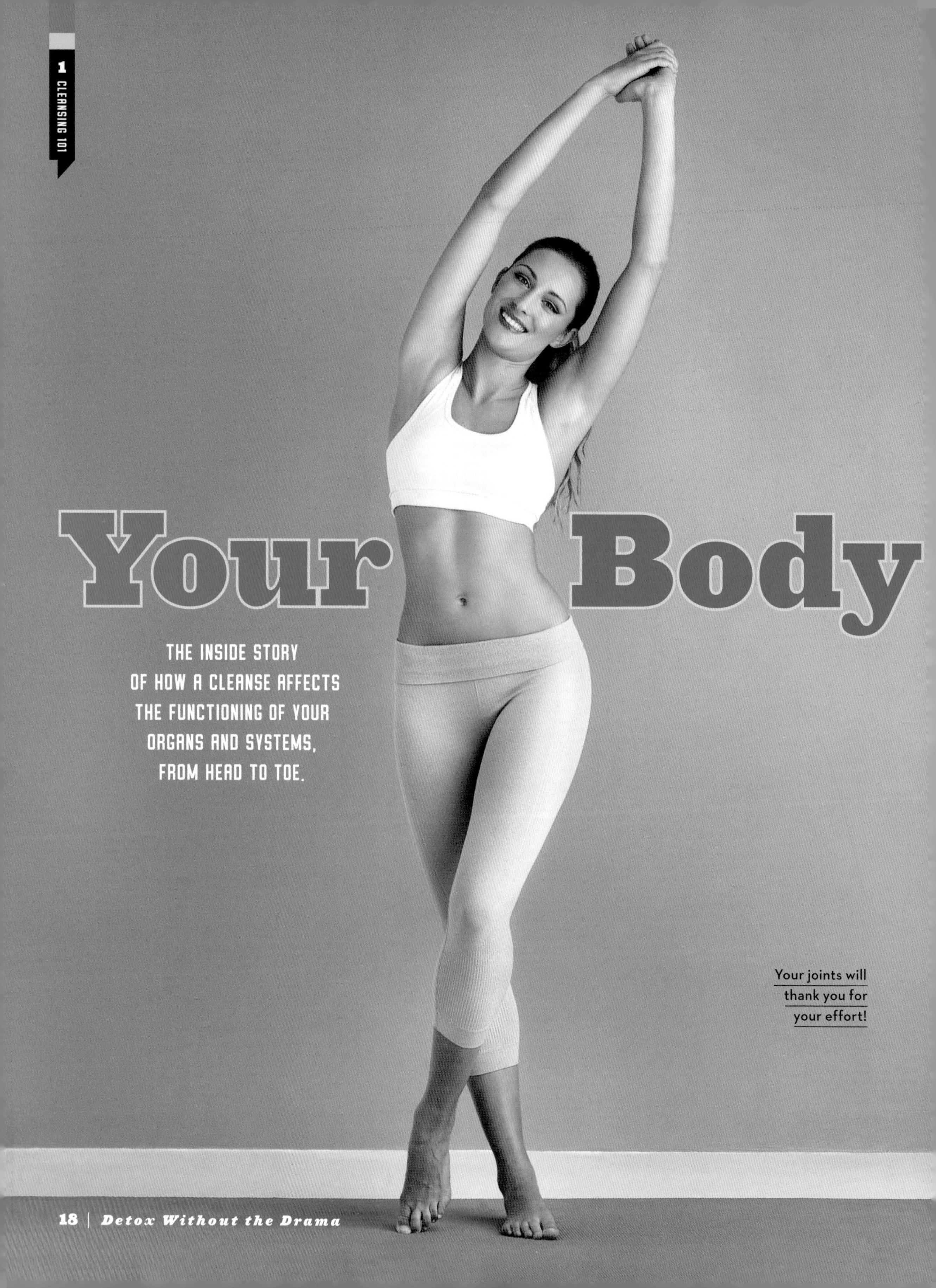

Your Body

THE INSIDE STORY
OF HOW A CLEANSE AFFECTS
THE FUNCTIONING OF YOUR
ORGANS AND SYSTEMS,
FROM HEAD TO TOE.

Your joints will
thank you for
your effort!

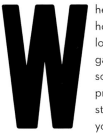

Whether you're hoping to lose weight, gain energy, solve digestive problems, strengthen your immune system—or all of the above—embarking on a cleanse will have profound effects on your body. It's like a spring-cleaning for your systems, says Peter Bennett, ND, co-author of *7-Day Detox Miracle*.

On a Detox

"Detoxification works because it addresses the needs of individual cells, the smallest units of human life," says Bennett. "It's the way the body heals itself, an internal cleansing process that takes place continuously." And you can help that process along, he says, by removing and eliminating toxins and supercharging every cell with healthy nutritional fuel—the definition of a detox or cleanse. "You change the oil in your car regularly," Bennett points out. "We recognize the need for exchanging old used fluids for new clean fluids in our mechanical world—but this idea hasn't translated into Western medicine." Once you decide to undertake that exchange through a cleanse or detox, here's what happens to your body.

Brain

The firing of neurons and synapses in the brain produces waste elements that must be cleared out—mostly during sleep, which is why improving your sleep quantity and quality is an important element of cleansing. Researchers have called sleep "the brain's garbage disposal system."

Lymph System

This network of tissues and organs is a key part of your body's immune system, working to remove dead or abnormal cells and foreign substances and transport lymph, a fluid full of infection-fighting white blood cells, throughout the body. "There are more lymph nodes in your intestines than anywhere else in your body," says Bennett, which is why cleanses focus on repairing gut function to strengthen the lymph system.

Lungs

The lungs are a key pathway for elimination, expelling toxins through exhalation. That's one reason why exercise, which raises both heart rate and oxygen uptake, plays such an important role in detoxing by speeding that elimination.

Liver

The liver is the heart of your natural detox system, says Bennett, it's "a massive processing center that not only breaks down nutrients such as fats and sugars from your foods, but also cleans the blood of the metabolic 'sweat,' or waste, of every cell in your body." Cleanses give your liver a rest from part of its processing work, so it can do a better job of cleaning your blood.

Pancreas

This organ produces insulin, a hormone that moves sugars from food out of the blood and into cells for fuel. The typical American diet, with its refined carbs and sugars, can lead to dysfunction in this system, in the form of both insulin resistance and Type 2 diabetes—both of which are skyrocketing in new cases. Cleanses reduce or eliminate dietary sugars, which help to give your pancreas a rest and help to normalize insulin function.

Body Fat

Most detoxes spur weight loss because they replace processed, unhealthy foods with fruits, vegetables and whole grains.

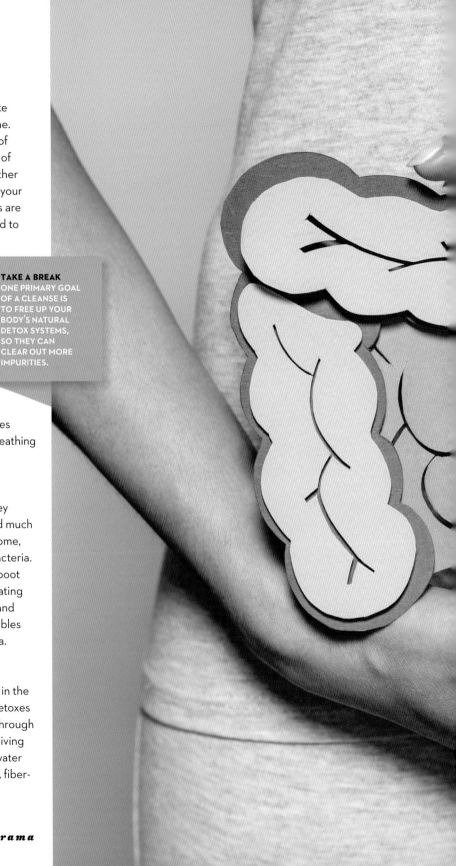

Kidneys

Your kidneys flush out waste and impurities through urine. Most cleanses involve lots of water, which helps dispose of toxins that your liver and other organs break down during your program. "Your body's cells are continuously being repaired to function optimally and break down nutrients," says Gavin Van De Walle, MS, RD, president of Dakota Dietitians. "These processes release wastes in the form of urea and carbon dioxide. Water transports these waste products and removes them through urination, breathing or sweating."

TAKE A BREAK ONE PRIMARY GOAL OF A CLEANSE IS TO FREE UP YOUR BODY'S NATURAL DETOX SYSTEMS, SO THEY CAN CLEAR OUT MORE IMPURITIES.

Small Intestine

The gut is emerging as a key player in overall health, and much of that involves its microbiome, or community of helpful bacteria. Cleanses can "reset" or reboot the microbiome through eating foods such as bone broth and fiber-rich fruits and vegetables that foster healthy gut flora.

Large Intestine

Your colon is the final step in the elimination process, and detoxes help improve its function through a combination of fasting (giving everything a rest), lots of water and a microbiome-friendly, fiber-filled diet.

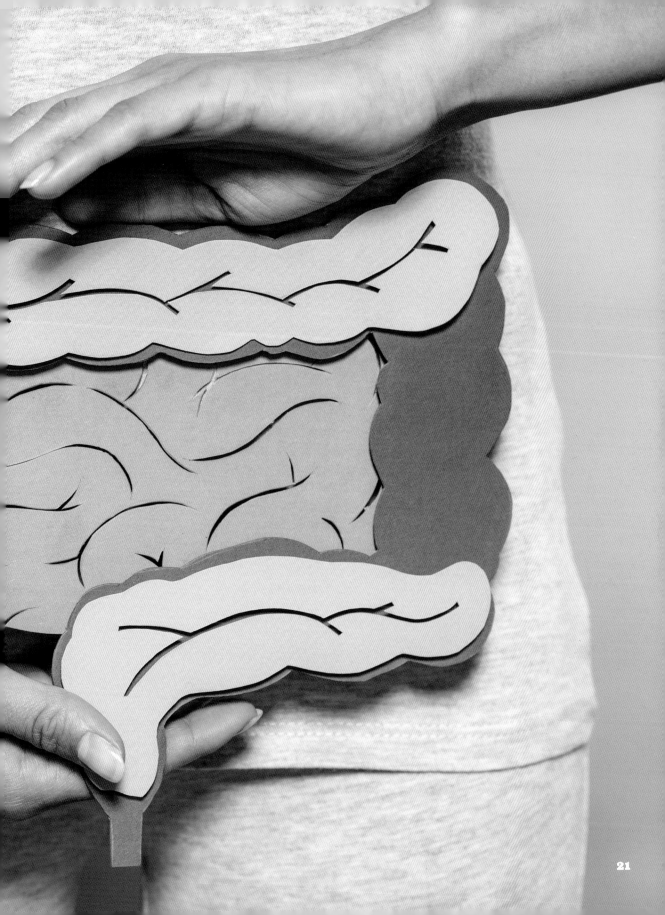

The Rich Tradition of Cleans

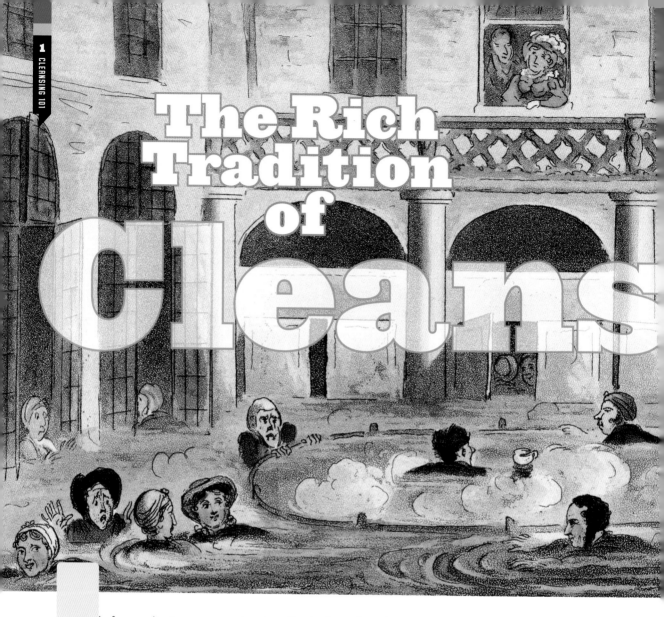

ong before medications were used to treat ailments ranging from an upset stomach to an infection, our ancestors looked to the natural world to restore health. While many modern cleanses focus on the intestinal microbiome and how it affects whole-body health, Hippocrates got there first—more than 2,000 years ago—when he said, "All disease begins in the gut."

"Every culture, every religion, has a form of enforced detoxification," says Peter Bennett, ND, co-author of *7-Day Detox Miracle*. "They all recognize that detoxification makes society healthier emotionally, physically and mentally." Take a tour through the history of this new-age "fad" that is rooted in thousands of years of traditional knowledge.

INDIA Ayurveda

Ayurveda is a holistic, mind-body philosophy that dates back more than 5,000 years. It emphasizes herbal treatments and bringing the body (and mind) into balance. A centerpiece of Ayurveda is *panchakarma* ("five actions"), a process of purification that includes steam therapy, lymphatic massage and herbal enemas. The aim is to cleanse the intestinal tract, purge toxins and rejuvenate the organs of elimination. "That sounds like the detoxes being done today," says Bennett.

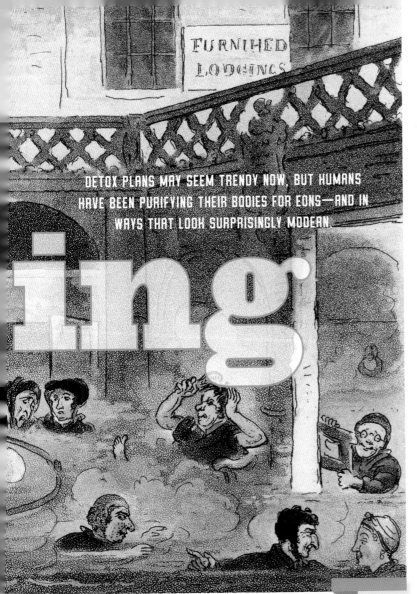

DETOX PLANS MAY SEEM TRENDY NOW, BUT HUMANS HAVE BEEN PURIFYING THEIR BODIES FOR EONS—AND IN WAYS THAT LOOK SURPRISINGLY MODERN

ing

just as sold on bathing rituals and have left ruins of bathhouses all over Europe. "Hydrotherapy has been employed for hundreds of years because of its ability to stimulate circulation," says Bennett.

THE AMERICAS
Native American Practices

Sweat lodges and fasting, two forms of detoxing, were mainstays of Native American cultures. Ancient tribes practiced sweat-bath ceremonies for purification. Fasting continues to be used in vision quests—as a way to connect to spirituality. And we now know that skin is as much an organ of detoxification as the kidneys.

UNITED STATES
Clean Living

In the 19th century, a fascination with cleansing and special diets (later dubbed "the clean living movement") led Rev. Sylvester Graham to invent a whole wheat health bread that became today's Graham cracker. And John Harvey Kellogg, a reform-minded doctor, built a sanitarium in Battle Creek, Michigan, that combined hydrotherapy, exercise, abstinence from alcohol, and colonics. He pinpointed the importance of intestinal bacteria to good health a century before modern science did—and forever changed breakfast with his creation of cornflakes.

CHINA Traditional Chinese Medicine

Also thousands of years old, the Chinese system puts an emphasis on the liver, the organ involved in removing toxins from your body, as well as overall cleansing through herbal remedies and other procedures including bodywork, acupuncture and nutritional therapies using herbs that support the liver to help strengthen the body's own systems.

ANCIENT GREECE AND ROME
Hydrotherapy

The Greeks recognized the health benefits of thermal-water therapy and invented what we think of today as a spa. In the seaside town of Loutraki (Greek for "bath," "bathhouse" or "spa"), about 50 miles west of Athens, visitors arrived from all over for the warm waters. Romans were

THE ENGLISH BATHED IN ROMAN RUINS.

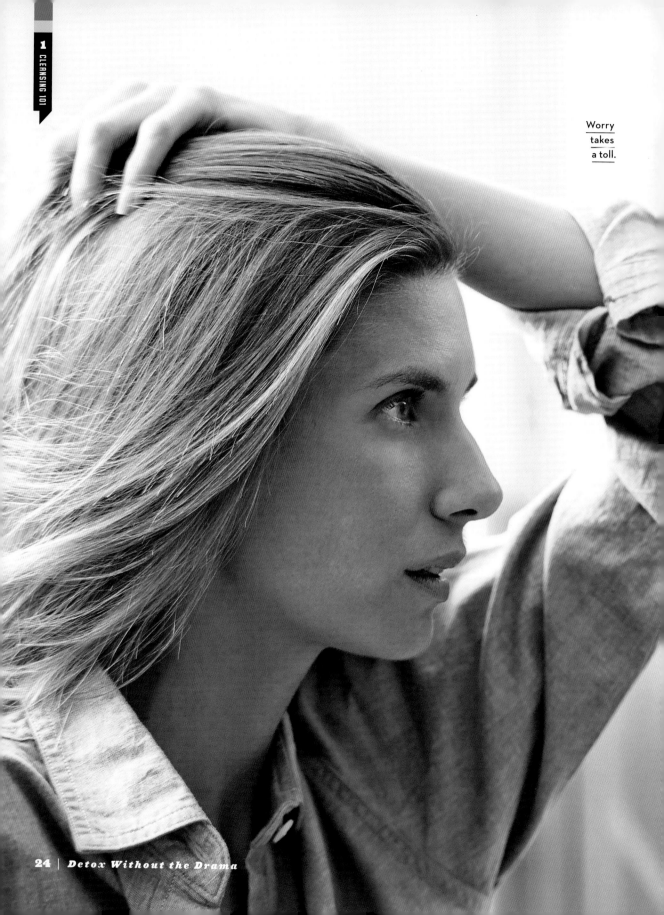

Worry
takes
a toll.

How Toxic Is Your Life?

FOOD-BASED CHEMICALS, POLLUTION, STRESS (AND STRESS-EATING OR DRINKING)—THE MODERN WORLD IS FILLED WITH HIDDEN HEALTH HAZARDS. USE THIS GUIDE TO DIAGNOSE YOUR STATUS.

There's no doubt about it: Our 21st-century lifestyle, and its conveniences, come with a cost. The cars and airplanes that whisk us around emit pollutants. Ready-made packaged foods are full of additives and preservatives. And our fast-paced, work-focused schedules can push stress to the front and exercise to the rear, with serious health consequences. "No one is free from the enormous amount of environmental and stress toxins assaulting us in our world," says Linda Page, ND, PhD, a naturopathic doctor and author of *Healthy Healing*. That's why virtually anyone can benefit from a cleanse. "It's one of the best ways to remain healthy in dangerous surroundings," says Page. "None of us is immune to environmental toxins, and most of us can't escape to a remote, unpolluted habitat."

If you're reading this and asking yourself, *Am I overdue for an intervention?*, think about how you feel right now. If you stop and really listen to your body, it will tell you how you're doing. Are you having trouble sleeping? Do you have digestive upsets often, such as nausea or constipation? How does your skin look—clear and fresh or blotchy and broken out? Is the number on the scale going up, even if you're trying to eat healthy? Other signs can include frequent headaches, back or joint pain, sinus problems and fatigue or brain fog, says Page. These are just a few ways your body can clue you in that it's time for a change. (For a complete checklist of symptoms, see page 28).

Next, do a mental inventory of your life—your habits, your behaviors, your surroundings and the products you use. "Even small changes in our environment can make a significant difference in our risk for development of disease," says Melissa Young, MD, an integrative and functional medicine specialist at the Cleveland Clinic. "You can decrease your exposure, for instance, by making better choices in food, beauty and cleaning products, and ventilating your home." Here's what to inventory:

CONSEQUENCES CANCER, OBESITY, NEUROLOGICAL DISEASES AND OTHER CONDITIONS HAVE BEEN LINKED TO TOXINS IN THE ENVIRONMENT.

Your Lifestyle

You make choices every day about how you live—and they all have an impact on your level of toxicity. First, consider what you eat. The more food you eat from a box, bag or freezer package, the more likely it is that you're carrying a toxic load. And it goes without saying that if you indulge in fast food, you're taking in unhealthy, highly processed fats, which become toxic at high heats. Even if you're eating whole foods, like lots of nutrient-dense produce in its original state, much of our food is grown with the aid of pesticides and fungicides. Choosing to buy organic can help lower your levels of these, says Young, especially if you prioritize buying organic versions of the most pesticide-filled foods (see the Environmental Working Group's "Dirty Dozen," a list of the top contaminated produce, at ewg.org). If you can't afford to buy exclusively organic fare, when you shop for, say, strawberries (they're at the very top of the list along with spinach and kale), grab the organic version.

Next, examine your "sins": alcohol, smoking, vaping and possibly even caffeine. There's a reason why we call the state of inebriation "intoxicated," because

Lower your *toxic load* one step at a time.

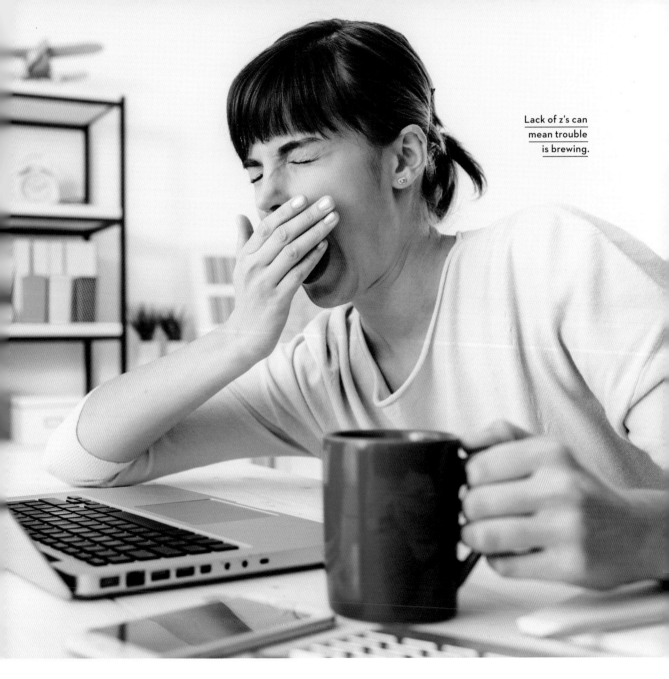

Lack of z's can mean trouble is brewing.

alcohol is literally a toxin. And the more of it you drink, the harder your liver—the primary detox organ—has to work, meaning that it may not be clearing out other toxins as efficiently because it's still working on last night's wine. Similarly, smoking hijacks another key organ that works to detox your body: your lungs. And although we don't know the full story on vaping yet, it's intuitive that inhaling an addictive substance into your lungs is a bad idea. Caffeine is a somewhat different animal, because many studies have shown benefits from coffee, for instance, which is a potent antioxidant. But again, it's an addictive substance, and most cleanses suggest clearing it out of your system, at least for a period of time.

Another powerful engine for detox is exercise, and there again many people fall short. If lack of time, motivation or energy

Toxicity Questionnaire

Take this detailed quiz to see where you stand—and chart your progress going forward.

This toxicity and symptom screening questionnaire covers symptoms that help to identify the underlying causes of illness and give you a sense of your level of overall toxicity. Rate each of the following symptoms based upon your health profile for the past 30 days.

POINT SCALE
0 = Never or almost never have the symptom. 1 = Occasionally have it, effect is not severe. 2 = Occasionally have it, effect is severe. 3 = Frequently have it, effect is not severe. 4 = Frequently have it, effect is severe.

HEAD
____ Headaches
____ Faintness
____ Dizziness
____ Insomnia
____ TOTAL

MOUTH/THROAT
____ Chronic coughing
____ Gagging/ frequent need to clear
____ Sore/hoarse/loss of voice
____ Swollen/discolored tongue/gum/lips
____ Canker sores
____ TOTAL

NOSE
____ Stuffy
____ Sinus problems
____ Hay fever
____ Sneezing attacks
____ Excessive mucus formation
____ TOTAL

EARS
____ Itchy
____ Earaches/ear infections
____ Drainage from ear
____ Ringing in ears/ hearing loss
____ TOTAL

EYES
____ Watery/itchy
____ Swollen/red/sticky eyelids
____ Bags or dark circles under eyes
____ Blurred or tunnel vision (does not include near- or farsightedness)
____ TOTAL

SKIN
____ Acne
____ Hives/rashes/dry skin
____ Hair loss
____ Flushing/hot flashes
____ Excessive sweating
____ TOTAL

HEART
____ Irregular/skipped heartbeat
____ Rapid/pounding heartbeat
____ Chest pain
____ TOTAL

LUNGS
____ Chest congestion
____ Asthma/bronchitis
____ Shortness of breath
____ Difficulty breathing
____ TOTAL

DIGESTIVE TRACT
____ Nausea/vomiting
____ Diarrhea
____ Constipation
____ Bloated feeling
____ Belching or passing gas
____ Heartburn
____ Intestinal/stomach pain
____ TOTAL

JOINTS/MUSCLES
____ Pains/aches in joints
____ Arthritis
____ Stiffness/limitation of movement
____ Pains/aches in muscles
____ Feeling of weakness/tiredness
____ TOTAL

EMOTIONS
____ Mood swings
____ Anxiety/fear/ nervousness
____ Anger/irritability/ aggressiveness
____ Depression
____ TOTAL

MIND
____ Poor memory
____ Confusion/poor comprehension
____ Poor concentration
____ Difficulty in making decisions
____ Stuttering/ stammering
____ Slurred speech
____ Learning disabilities
____ TOTAL

ENERGY/ACTIVITY

_____ Fatigue/
   sluggishness
_____ Apathy/lethargy
_____ Hyperactivity
_____ Restlessness
_____ **TOTAL**

WEIGHT

_____ Binge eating/
   drinking
_____ Craving certain
   foods
_____ Overweight
_____ Compulsive eating
_____ Water retention
_____ Underweight
_____ **TOTAL**

OTHER

_____ Frequent illness
_____ Frequent/urgent
   urination
_____ Genital itch
_____ **TOTAL**

GRAND TOTAL

Add up the individual points to reach a score for each group. Add the group scores together to get a grand total.

Less than 10: Optimal. 10–50: Mild Toxicity. 50–100: Moderate Toxicity. Over 100: Severe Toxicity.

has led you into a sedentary (aka couch potato) existence, your body doesn't get a chance to lower inflammation—a key driver of systemic toxicity—and expel toxins through sweat and exhalation. Not to mention the many ways exercise can reduce your stress level and benefit your body as a whole.

Your Environment

When it comes to how toxic your surroundings are, certain things are at least partly out of your control. For instance, if you live in a ground-floor apartment on a heavily traveled city street, you're breathing air that is likely full of particles from various sources. If you live in a small town in rural Georgia or Montana, the air outside is probably considerably cleaner—unless there's a massive power plant nearby.

That said, your indoor environment is in many ways modifiable. Young actually advises opening your windows frequently no matter where you live, because, she says, "indoor air pollution is significantly higher than outdoor air pollution." That's especially true if you're a fan of air fresheners, if you like using powerful commercial cleaning products full of bleach or ammonia—and even if you're not a very avid cleaner. For instance, Young says, "pesticides and allergens are carried in dust," so you should dust your space weekly—but not by using a spray,

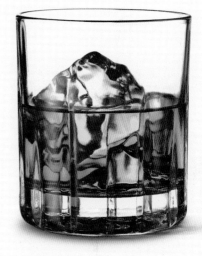

which releases its own load of toxins into the air.

Go look under your kitchen sink. If it's packed with conventional cleaners, you may have built-up toxins in your system. Open your makeup bag and medicine chest. See a collection of perfumed lotions and conventionally made foundation, eye shadow and mascara? "Endocrine disrupters such as phthalates, parabens and BPA are widely found in personal beauty products and cleaning products," says Young.

What's the verdict? No matter how careful you are, your body is inevitably exposed to the toxins—and, sometimes, toxic lifestyles—inherent in the modern world. This book will help you treat your mind and body to a deep cleaning.

29

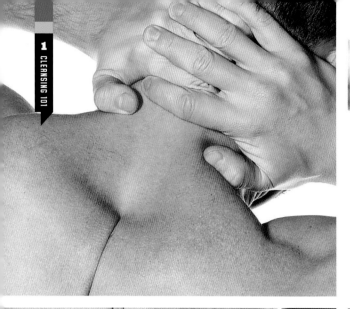
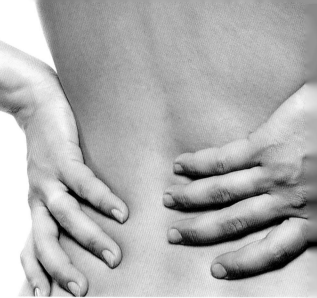
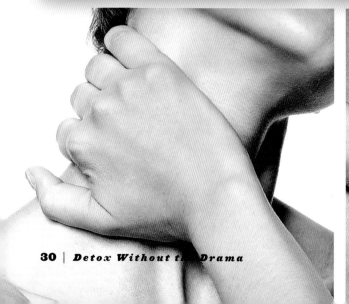

Target: Inflam

THIS POWERFUL INTERNAL FORCE—
FOR BOTH GOOD AND BAD—IS AT THE
HEART OF MANY OF THE ILLS THAT PROMPT
A DETOX. HERE'S HOW IT WORKS, AND WHY
A CLEANSE CAN CALM THE FLAMES.

f you could use only two words to describe the most important goal of a detox, it would likely be "reduce inflammation." That's because chronic inflammation has emerged as a key player in all kinds of dysfunction inside the body, from heart disease to dementia to diabetes to digestive issues and immune disorders. A major study published in the journal *Nature Medicine* found that diseases linked to chronic inflammation are "the most significant cause of death in the world today," accounting for more than 50% of global deaths. The connection between inflammation and physical and mental decline is so strong that researchers have invented a term—"inflammaging"—

changes, exercise, sleep and stress reduction, can reduce inflammation. Read on for a short course in quieting your inflammatory response.

What Is Inflammation?

At its heart, inflammation is a protective response your body mounts to a threat. Think of the redness that develops around a cut or scrape, or the swelling and feeling of heat around a sprained ankle. This is acute inflammation: Your body is sending white blood cells to the site of an injury to prevent further damage, promote healing, and fight infection. It's a sign that your inner workings are on high

But things get tricky when inflammation lingers too long, she adds. "As the body's response shifts from acute to chronic, the inflammatory machinery takes a different tack, one that results in progressive tissue damage rather than repair."

That's because some of the proteins and hormones that are released in response to acute injury or stress can become toxic to various parts of your body. For instance, the stress hormone cortisol is released in a fight-or-flight scenario and helps you escape danger by flooding your body with glucose (including inhibiting insulin production to keep the glucose circulating) and narrowing the arteries, while

mation

to refer to inflammation's role in how healthfully (or not) you age.

It's not just inflammation's physical toll that makes it a target of detox, though—it's also that inflammation is highly amenable to lifestyle changes, especially the kinds that happen with a cleanse. In fact, all of the strategies you're reading about in this book, including dietary

alert, alarm bells are ringing, and your cells are laboring to fix the injury. Neuropsychiatrist Louann Brizendine, MD, calls this process "a beautifully choreographed dance performed by the immune system in our bodies and brains. When sparked by an injury, infection or other insult, the body creates an acute inflammatory cascade to quickly repair tissues."

epinephrine, another stress hormone, increases the heart rate, both of which force blood to pump harder and faster. All of these actions are harmful in the long term—leading to blood-sugar imbalance and potentially diabetes, weight gain (because of its effects on insulin functioning, cortisol also increases appetite), immune-system suppression, high blood pressure, heart damage, and compromised digestion (which can lead to leaky gut syndrome, in which toxins can leak out of the intestines into nearby tissues and organs).

Also released during chronic inflammatory response are proteins known as cytokines, which spring into action when your body or brain is injured, traumatized or under chronic stress, says Brizendine. "They're like messengers zipping around, alerting your immune system to get moving and deal with the threat." But when they're being released constantly, cytokines can have unintended consequences. "For example, cytokines have been shown to disrupt the release of neurotransmitters, including serotonin and dopamine, two essential 'feel-good' chemicals," says Brizendine. "That's the opposite of what antidepressants do," hence the role of stress and inflammation in promoting anxiety and depression.

What Causes It?

Chronic inflammation can be the result of emotional stress, but also of many physical factors: certain diets, a sedentary lifestyle, lack of sleep and others. The following checklist shows the major offenders—and also serves as an introduction to the ways this book can help you prevent and reduce inflammation through a healthy detox program.

Stress

Feeling overwhelmed or over tasked for extended periods of time fires up chemicals that, as described earlier, can have far-reaching consequences for your body and brain. And these effects can become self-perpetuating. "A 2019 study showed that high markers of inflammation predicted worsening mood symptoms of depression," says Brizendine. "Then that cycle keeps going, because a lack of positive mood also predicted increasing inflammation over time." **To Fix It** See page 72 for an explanation of how yoga can help you de-stress, and page 84 for advice on meditation.

DOUBLE-EDGED SWORD INFLAMMATION IS LITERALLY A LIFE-SAVER—UNTIL IT BECOMES A THREAT. A CLEANSE CAN LOWER THE RISKS.

Unhealthy Diet

What you eat has a huge effect on inflammation, which is one main reason that detoxes and cleanses focus so much on foods and dietary plans. First, processed foods in general have been strongly linked to raising inflammation, because they're typically loaded with ingredients that have been shown to be highly inflammatory in studies. These can include added sugars, unhealthy types of fats (such as trans fats) and highly refined

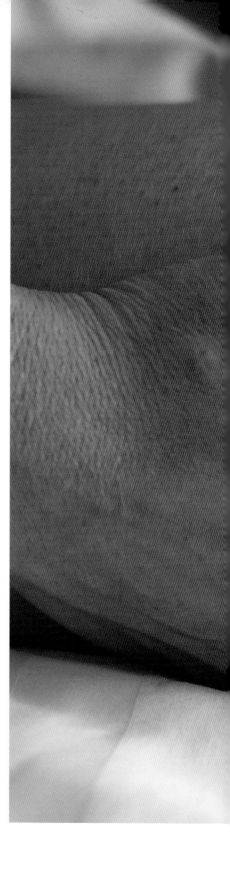

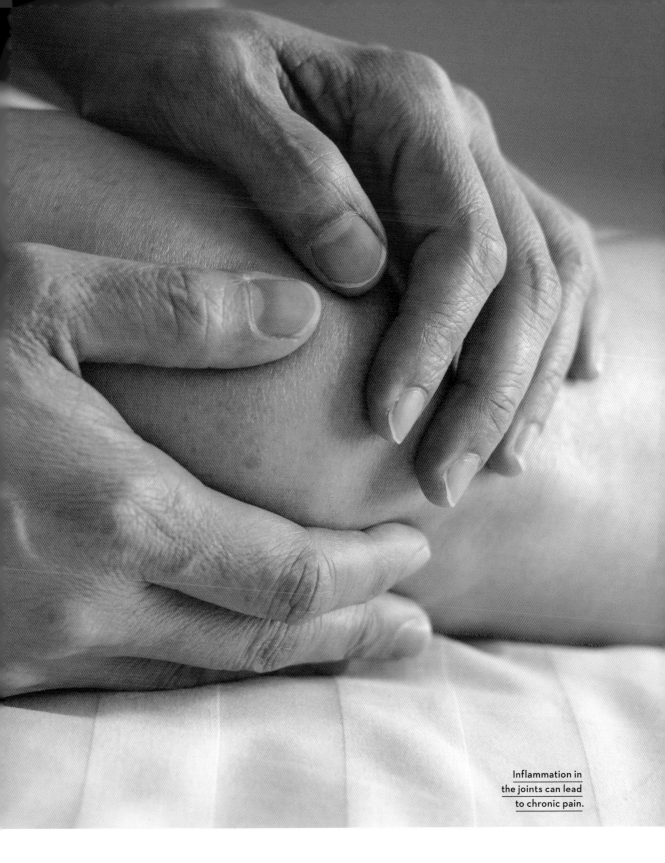

Inflammation in
the joints can lead
to chronic pain.

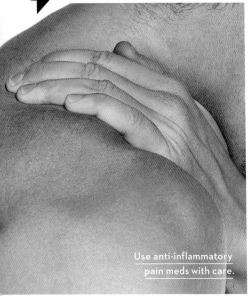

Use anti-inflammatory
pain meds with care.

of inflammation. **To Fix It** See page 92 for a comprehensive list of anti-inflammatory and detoxing foods, and the recipes starting on page 150 for healthy inspiration.

Lack of Exercise
Being sedentary is a national epidemic, but working out—despite temporarily stressing your body—is a powerful anti-inflammatory tool. Whether or not it helps you to lose weight, exercise has been shown to lower multiple pro-inflammatory molecules and cytokines. A study in the journal *Brain, Behavior, and Immunity* found that a single

amounts of adipokines, which are inflammatory cytokines that influence the immune system." There is also evidence that insulin resistance, common among the overweight, can cause more inflammatory cytokines to circulate in the body. And once you do have chronic inflammation, it can work to keep you overweight by further impairing your insulin response, leading to even more weight gain. **To Fix It** All of the strategies in this book—from eating better to exercising to reducing stress and environmental toxins—will aid in losing weight.

carbohydrates, all of which raise inflammatory markers, trigger an immune response and suppress the "good" bacteria in your gut microbiome. A meat-heavy diet high in saturated fat also promotes inflammation. "Just having a single can of soda has been shown to increase inflammatory markers in the blood," says Naomi Whittel, author of *High Fiber Keto*. When you replace these with fresh, real, whole foods—fish, whole grains and lots of produce—you'll not only be taking in a raft of anti-inflammatory nutrients, phytochemicals and vitamins, but you'll also be feeding that helpful bacteria. This basically describes the Mediterranean diet, which a study in the journal *Nutrients* (among many others) has found may lower markers

Use your body's *protection* well.

20-minute exercise session produces an anti-inflammatory response and also prompts a release of hormones, such as epinephrine and norepinephrine, that activate immune-cell receptors. **To Fix It** Turn to page 66 for advice on how to ramp up your activity.

Obesity
Carrying too much weight is a double whammy: It is both a cause and an effect of inflammation. If you're overweight, says Whittel, "it may be that adipose tissue is releasing increased

Inadequate Sleep
Not getting enough quality z's can prompt inflammatory changes throughout the body. A study in the journal *Biological Psychiatry* found that just one bad night's sleep can trigger key cellular pathways that fuel inflammation. Other studies have shown that good sleep, on the other hand, strengthens the immune system and helps dysregulate inflammatory and antiviral responses. **To Fix It** See page 54 for a guide to the best detoxing sleep strategies.

Top Hot Spots in Your Body

The impact is widespread, affecting key organs that are involved in detoxing.

HEART Inflammation is emerging as a key factor in cardiovascular disease, as it appears to damage the interior of blood vessels, promote the growth of plaque that can narrow arteries and also loosen plaque, which can trigger blood clots—the primary cause of heart attacks and strokes.

LIVER Chronic inflammation can cause an enlarged liver or fatty liver disease, resulting in an increased toxic load buildup throughout the body. Since the liver is your primary detoxing organ, this is especially worrisome for your future health (and a reason that all cleanses and detoxes emphasize rehabilitating the liver).

JOINTS Arthritis and other joint pain and diseases are closely linked to inflammation, which attacks joint tissues and can cause swelling, increased joint fluid, cartilage and bone damage, and muscle loss. Lowering inflammation levels can help prevent or treat joint issues.

BRAIN Systemic inflammation can cause depression, brain fog and even increase the risk of dementia. Inflammatory cytokines that are released during ongoing stress can reduce the number of protective proteins in the brain—proteins that normally encourage growth of new neurons and synapses in the parts of the brain that handle learning, memory and higher thinking.

PANCREAS Your pancreas is the source of insulin, so when chronic inflammation increases your body's insulin resistance, the pancreas has to work harder. When the pancreas can't keep up, it can lead to Type 2 diabetes.

GUT Many digestive diseases, such as irritable bowel syndrome, Crohn's disease and celiac disease, are linked to inflammation, which can damage the intestinal lining and precede leaky gut syndrome. In that case, toxins can "leak" directly from your intestines into your bloodstream.

SKIN Many skin conditions—including rashes, dermatitis, eczema, acne and psoriasis—can be traced to chronic inflammation (one reason a detox can give you clearer, healthier skin).

JLo got her glow on for the 2020 Super Bowl.

Jennifer Lopez

To prepare for her triumphant 2020 Super Bowl LIV performance, the singer/dancer/actor went on a restrictive diet created by trainer to the stars Tracy Anderson. Dubbed "JLo's 10-Day No-Sugar No-Carb Challenge," the plan eliminated all sugar, including fruit, grains and alcohol, and stuck to a menu of lean proteins, eggs, avocado, non-starchy veggies, nuts and seeds. Although Lopez says she was "hungry all the time," that halftime show proved her efforts paid off.

Celebrity Detox

NO, NOT *THAT* KIND OF DETOX! THE RICH, FAMOUS AND GLAMOROUS HAVE JUMPED ON THE CLEANSING BANDWAGON, BIG-TIME.

The word "detox" has taken on a whole new meaning in Hollywood and on red carpets everywhere. Celebs are often on the cutting edge of health trends—especially when the benefits include weight loss. Whether it's to refresh the system after a demanding project, or to prep for a cover shoot or performance, high-profile insiders are swapping out substances such as caffeine and sugar for juices and "clean" food. From Salma Hayek's juice cleanse to Gwyneth Paltrow's 7-Day Detox, here are the top ways A-listers have been resetting their bodies and regaining their energy.

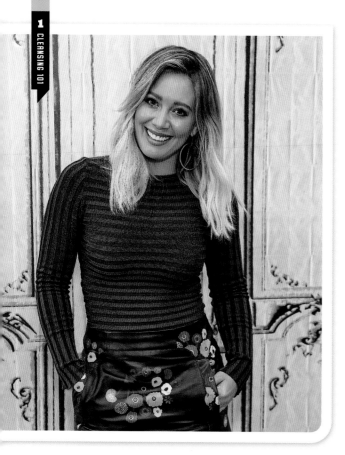

Salma Hayek

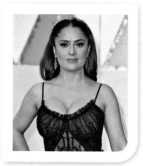

The Mexican-born actor is famous for her sexy, voluptuous figure, but even she depends on a healthy cleanse to hit the reset button every now and then. Together with Juice Generation's Eric Helms, Hayek created a line of detoxifying drinks, now known as the Cooler Cleanse. You can choose among different plans, from Juice for a Day to the 5-Day Cleanse. "It's like my meditation," says Hayek. "It makes me stop, focus and think about what I'm putting into my body. I'm making a commitment to my health."

Hilary Duff

To promote circulation and detoxify the liver, celebrities such as supermodel Heidi Klum and actor Jennifer Aniston down a daily dose of apple cider vinegar, either diluted in water or as part of a dressing for their salads. But *Younger* actor Hilary Duff is strictly hard-core in her love of the sour liquid. "I'll just shoot it straight in the morning," says the mother of two. "People think it's gross, but I kind of like the taste."

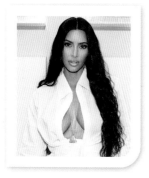

Kim Kardashian

Whenever the fashion/lifestyle influencer needs to drop a few pounds stat, like for the annual Met Gala, she turns to the Sunfare Optimal Cleanse, a 10-day detox that is available online. The program includes shakes, organic proteins and veggies, and wild-caught fish. A typical day: three "Cleanse" shakes, turkey chili, grilled salmon with millet pilaf and no refined sugar. "I wanted to just change my food patterns," says Kardashian. "I wanted to eat healthier and cut sugar out of my life as much as I can."

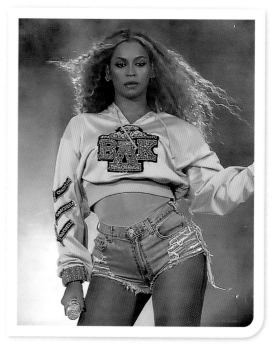

Beyoncé

When the singer/songwriter/dancer and multi-Grammy winner was preparing for her historic 2018 Coachella performance, she had just given birth to twins and weighed around 175 pounds. Determined to be in her best shape, she turned to friend, trainer and exercise physiologist Marco Borges to help her drop weight and reboot her body with the 22 Days Nutrition diet. The plan consists of fruit, veggies, whole grains and seeds. And yes, "lemonade"-infused water for the *Lemonade* star!

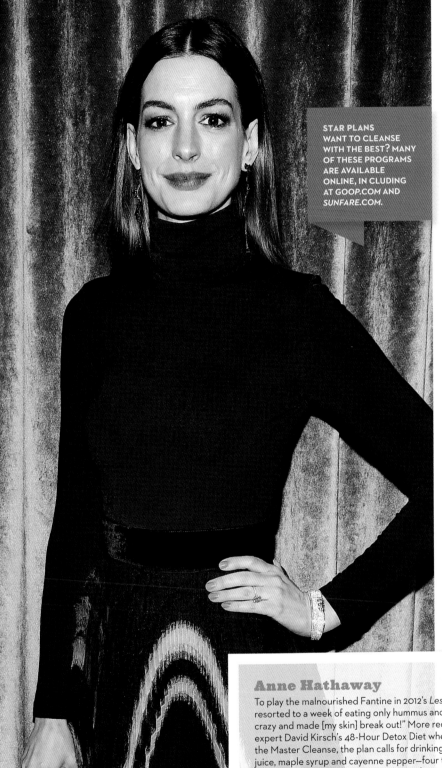

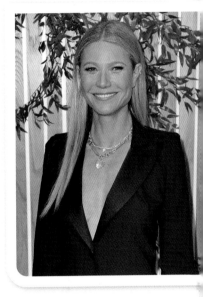

Gwyneth Paltrow

"I created the 7-Day Detox as an elimination diet," the Oscar winner wrote on her Goop blog. A cleansing expert who likes to fast and detox a couple of times a year, Paltrow's weeklong meal plan consists of beet-carrot-apple-ginger juices, green smoothies, salads, soups, fruits, seeds and nuts, lean proteins such as fish and chicken, and whole grains. Now we know how she's managed to maintain her slim figure and natural glow.

Anne Hathaway

To play the malnourished Fantine in 2012's *Les Misérables*, the Oscar winner resorted to a week of eating only hummus and radishes, adding that the diet "was crazy and made [my skin] break out!" More recently, she has turned to fitness expert David Kirsch's 48-Hour Detox Diet when she needs a reboot. Much like the Master Cleanse, the plan calls for drinking a formula called LemonAid—lemon juice, maple syrup and cayenne pepper—four times per day for two days. It's considered extreme by many health professionals, but most agree that a short-term cleanse will eliminate toxins and aid in quick weight loss.

Celebrity Retreats

Luxury wellness spas have long been hot spots for the rich and famous. From destination desert retreats with yoga and meditation to full-on diet detox centers serving pure juices and spa cuisine, here are three worth saving up for.

MIRAVAL SPA, TUCSON, ARIZONA

Set in the majestic Santa Catalina Mountains, this all-inclusive resort's mission is to inspire each person to create a life in balance. One of Oprah Winfrey's favorite getaways, Miraval offers a full menu of yoga, meditation, hydrotherapy, hiking and equine therapy. But you know if Oprah loves it, there has to be incredible spa food, too. Not only do they serve guests organic, palate-pleasing meals, but they also offer a variety of cuisine-based workshops covering anti-inflammatory foods, plant-based cooking and recipes for a healthy gut.

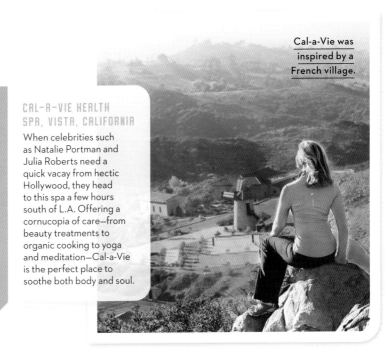

Cal-a-Vie was inspired by a French village.

CAL-A-VIE HEALTH SPA, VISTA, CALIFORNIA

When celebrities such as Natalie Portman and Julia Roberts need a quick vacay from hectic Hollywood, they head to this spa a few hours south of L.A. Offering a cornucopia of care—from beauty treatments to organic cooking to yoga and meditation—Cal-a-Vie is the perfect place to soothe both body and soul.

WE CARE SPA, COACHELLA VALLEY, CALIFORNIA

Located in Desert Hot Springs, California, this retreat is a leader in juice fasting and colonics. Stars such as Matthew McConaughey, Ben Affleck and Gwen Stefani have been seen lounging around the pool and gardens of this detoxification desert spa. During their stay, guests follow a liquid diet of organic juices and smoothies, and choose from treatments such as body wraps, facials, colonics and massages designed to enhance the fast's detoxifying effects. Classes in food prep, yoga and healing are offered to help keep guests in the detox zone long after they return home.

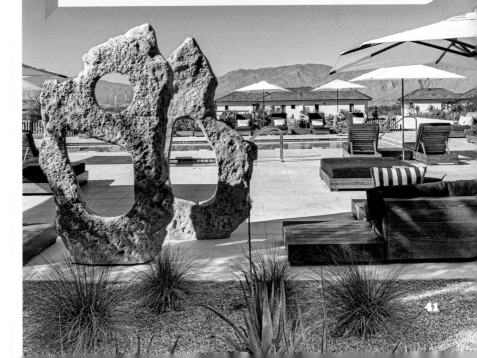

Say "ah" with an Ayurvedic herbal-oil massage.

41

DIY Detox Retreats

Want all the benefits of a spa without breaking the bank? Here are some inexpensive at-home tips to get your mind, body and spirit back on track.

Studies show being outdoors is calming.

TAKE A HIKE

Walking those famous 10,000 steps is one of America's favorite ways to stay in shape. Not only is it key to maintaining a healthy body weight, but it also helps lower blood pressure, and just being in nature has been shown to lift your mood. But what exactly is the difference between a walk and hike? According to Gregory Miller, former president of the American Hiking Society, a hike—whether it's on a wilderness trail or a paved city sidewalk in an urban landscape—is when you're walking for fun or fitness and enjoying the view and the journey you're on. His advice: "Find a nearby trail, take a hike and experience the natural wonders of a city park or the backcountry wilderness." Check out americanhiking.org for information on trails near you.

DITCH YOUR DEVICES

Whether you're going on vacation or having a staycation, putting away all your screens for a period of time—say, one or two days—can be hugely freeing. Does that sound like a lot of time? Singer Selena Gomez told *US Weekly* that she went cold turkey without her cell phone for three months. "It was the most refreshing, calming, rejuvenating feeling," she said. And studies show that being connected to tech 24/7 can be bad for your physical and mental health. For more on doing your own digital detox, see page 89.

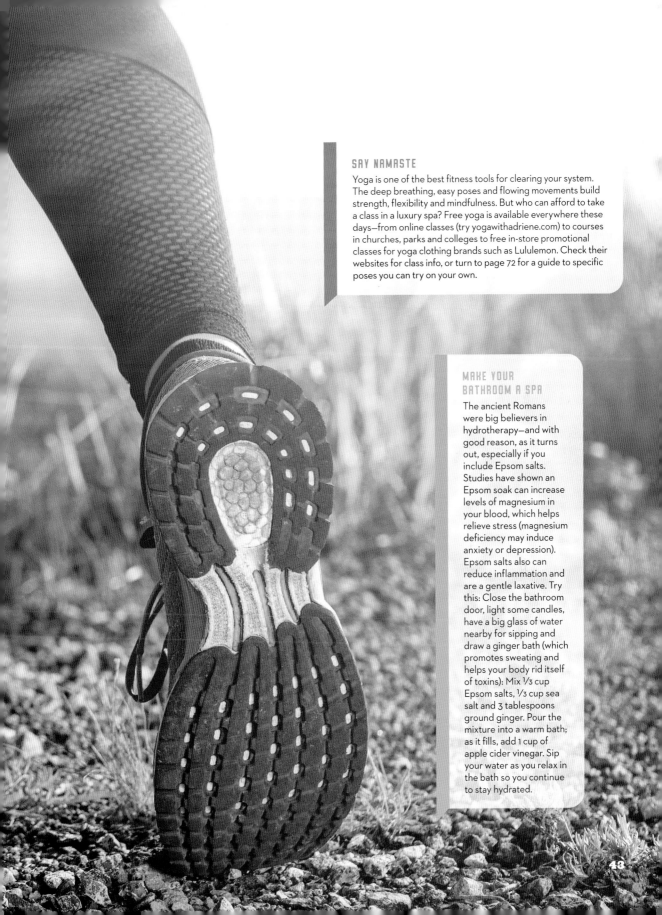

SAY NAMASTE

Yoga is one of the best fitness tools for clearing your system. The deep breathing, easy poses and flowing movements build strength, flexibility and mindfulness. But who can afford to take a class in a luxury spa? Free yoga is available everywhere these days—from online classes (try yogawithadriene.com) to courses in churches, parks and colleges to free in-store promotional classes for yoga clothing brands such as Lululemon. Check their websites for class info, or turn to page 72 for a guide to specific poses you can try on your own.

MAKE YOUR BATHROOM A SPA

The ancient Romans were big believers in hydrotherapy—and with good reason, as it turns out, especially if you include Epsom salts. Studies have shown an Epsom soak can increase levels of magnesium in your blood, which helps relieve stress (magnesium deficiency may induce anxiety or depression). Epsom salts also can reduce inflammation and are a gentle laxative. Try this: Close the bathroom door, light some candles, have a big glass of water nearby for sipping and draw a ginger bath (which promotes sweating and helps your body rid itself of toxins): Mix 1/3 cup Epsom salts, 1/3 cup sea salt and 3 tablespoons ground ginger. Pour the mixture into a warm bath; as it fills, add 1 cup of apple cider vinegar. Sip your water as you relax in the bath so you continue to stay hydrated.

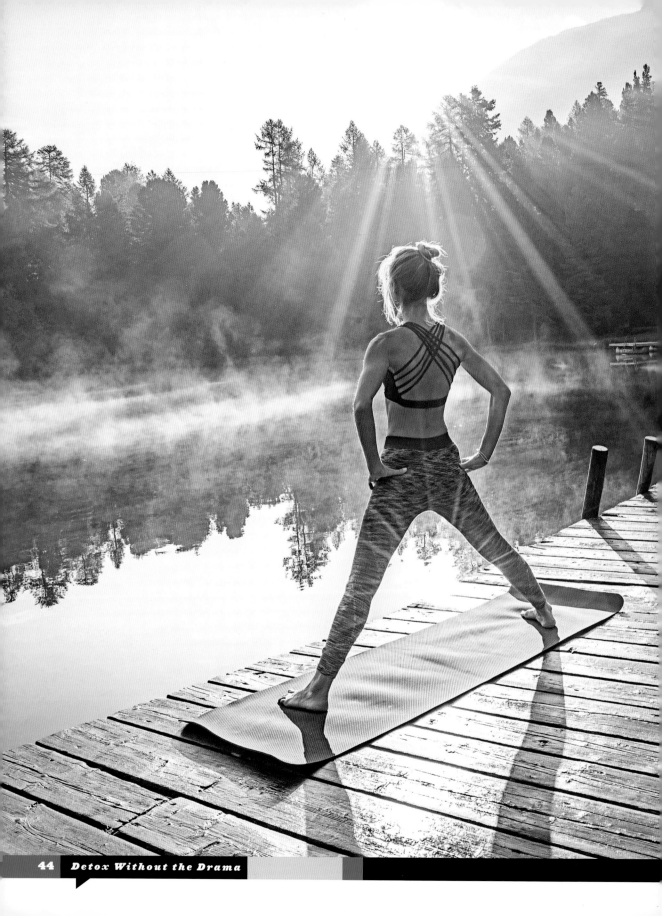

2

DETOX YOUR LIFESTYLE

FROM CONQUERING STRESS AND ENVIRONMENTAL TOXINS TO FIXING SLEEP AND EXERCISE HABITS, HERE'S HOW TO LIVE CLEANER.

Clean

IT'S NOT JUST ABOUT PURIFYING YOUR INTERNAL ENVIRONMENT. YOUR DAY-TO-DAY SURROUNDINGS CONTRIBUTE TO YOUR TOXIC LOAD—AND CLEANING THEM THE RIGHT WAY IS KEY.

t's no secret that city air can be polluted, streams may be rendered impotable by chemical runoff, and that conventionally farmed foods contain pesticide residues. But we tend to think of our homes as a refuge from these ambient toxicants, a place where we know to wash our produce and where we can let down our hair.

Unfortunately, it's not quite that simple, says Melissa Young, MD, an integrative and functional medicine specialist at the Cleveland Clinic. "There are toxins in our food supply and our air, in beauty products and household cleaners and in household items such as furniture, particle board, bedding and mattresses," says Young. Between air fresheners and mold and dust-mite dander and vinyl shower curtains that release volatile organic compounds (VOCs), your home sweet home is harboring loads of allergens, pollutants and toxins.

Environmental toxins have been associated with increased risk of insulin resistance, diabetes, heart disease, obesity and asthma, says Young. They're also associated with infertility and reproductive problems, as well as cancer and immune suppression. Add to that list pernicious but less easily

Dust often to
clear allergens
and toxins out.

House

SAFER SUDS
IN PLACE OF
COMMERCIAL
CLEANSERS, YOU
CAN USE A MIXTURE
OF BAKING SODA,
LEMON AND SALT
FOR CLEANING.

diagnosed conditions such as leaky gut syndrome. And there's another aspect of environmental toxins to consider: The more you are exposed to additional toxins, whether from medication, alcohol or chemicals in beauty products, cleaning products and household items, the harder your body (especially your liver) must work to detoxify not only those substances but also the more ordinary day-to-day toxins that you regularly encounter.

But there are things you can do to greatly lower your exposure inside your home—which, after all, is where you spend a good deal of your time each day—and these strategies should form a part of your overall detox or cleanse. "There is no way to completely avoid exposure to toxins, but you can absolutely make choices every day to decrease your exposure," says Young. Room by room, here's what you need to know—and do—to give your home its own cleanse.

Living Room

First and foremost, there's a very easily accomplished rule, advises Young: Take off your shoes when you enter your home. "Most household dirt, pesticides and lead come into your house on your shoes," she says. Also plan on opening your windows frequently to ventilate the entire space; especially in newer buildings that are more airtight, often the air outside (even if polluted by car fumes) is cleaner than your home's air. Worried about smells (last night's fish fry)? Opening your windows (if you don't live near a busy road) is better than using air fresheners. "They tend to be petroleum-based and contain endocrine disrupters," says Young.

You should also dust at least once a week, according to Young, "as pesticides and allergens are carried in dust." Instead of using a commercial spray (which can add to your chemical load) or feathers (which just spread more dust), use dry unscented microfiber cloths—they attract dirt particles instead of scattering them. To keep indoor air clean, consider buying an air purifier with a HEPA filter, which screens out very small particles of allergens, mold spores and other irritants.

Vacuums with HEPA filters are also the gold standard for scooping up microscopic particles. Hardwood floors are better than carpeting because they don't collect as many

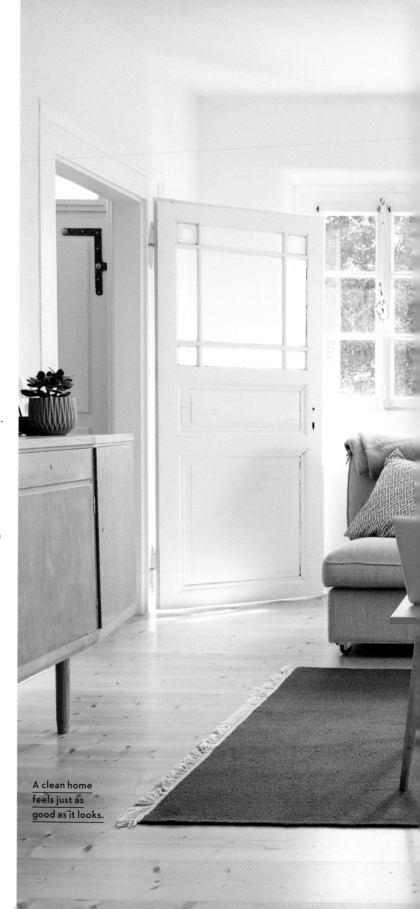

A clean home feels just as good as it looks.

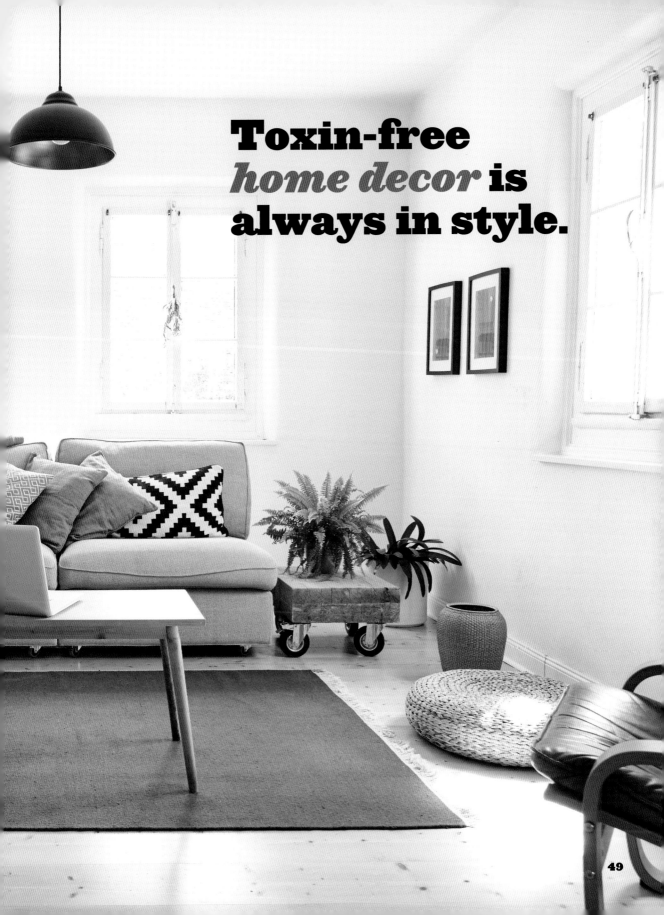

Toxin-free *home decor* is always in style.

Detox Your Digs

Map out a strategy to lower your home's toxic footprint.

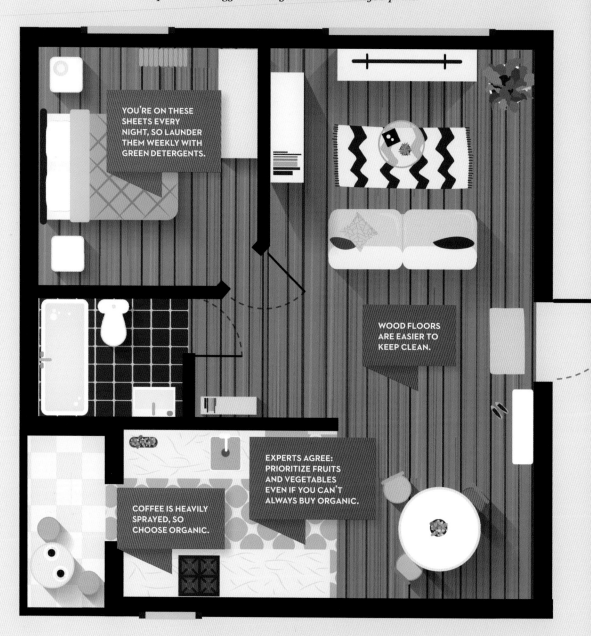

YOU'RE ON THESE SHEETS EVERY NIGHT, SO LAUNDER THEM WEEKLY WITH GREEN DETERGENTS.

WOOD FLOORS ARE EASIER TO KEEP CLEAN.

EXPERTS AGREE: PRIORITIZE FRUITS AND VEGETABLES EVEN IF YOU CAN'T ALWAYS BUY ORGANIC.

COFFEE IS HEAVILY SPRAYED, SO CHOOSE ORGANIC.

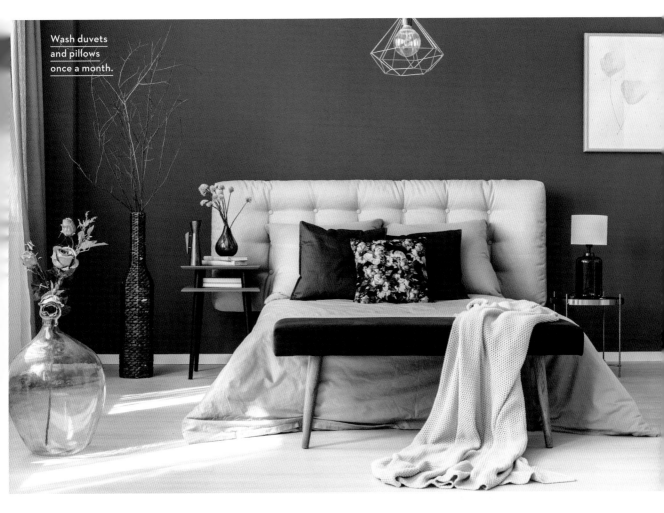

Wash duvets and pillows once a month.

particles (and some carpets may have synthetic coatings that release VOCs). If you're hoping that houseplants can clear the air of toxins—as has often been touted—studies show the effect is negligible.

Bedroom

Many of the toxin issues here are similar to the living room, with one big difference: This is likely the room where you spend the most number of hours, as it's where you sleep. So it's important to keep up regular dusting and vacuuming, and perhaps consider an air filter in the bedroom as well.

Bedding can be a source of many noxious substances, so cover your box spring, mattress and pillows in allergen-proof, airtight zippered covers (the Environmental Working Group, or EWG, recommends one made of a tightly woven fabric, such as cotton, instead of PVC or vinyl). Your mattress itself can be a source of contaminants and chemicals. The EWG suggests shopping for these criteria: no less than 95% organic content, no polyurethane foam, no added chemical flame retardants, low-VOC certification, no added fragrances or antimicrobials and no PVC or vinyl.

Wash bedding weekly in hot water and tumble dry, and look

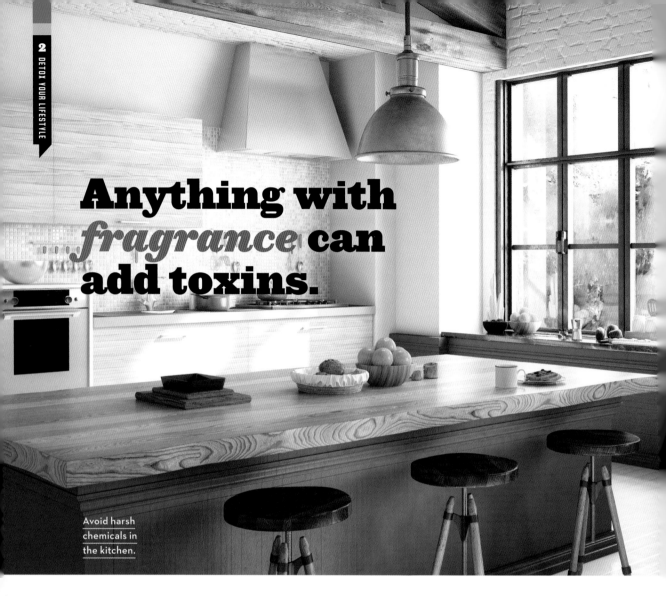

Anything with *fragrance* can add toxins.

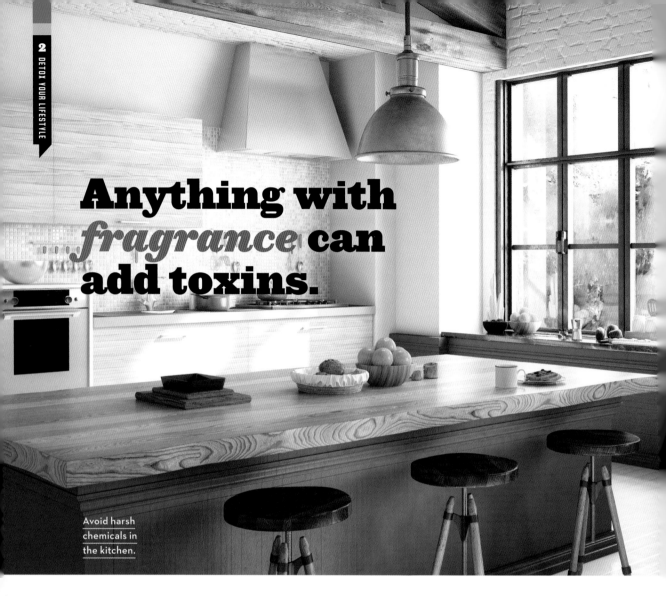

Avoid harsh chemicals in the kitchen.

for green laundry-detergent brands that are unscented (scents may trigger allergies and can contain endocrine disrupters). Look for products certified by Green Seal or EcoLogo; the EWG recommends the AspenClean brand. And those dryer sheets, like Bounce? Bounce 'em! Most brands coat fabric with chemicals such as quaternary ammonium compounds—which are linked to asthma—and acetone, the main ingredient in nail polish remover.

Kitchen

Many kitchen and bathroom cleaners contain toxic substances: Tile or sink cleansers can have ammonia or bleach, dish detergent may contain VOCs or carcinogens, sprays can promote asthma. The EWG tested 21 commonly used cleaning products—such as air fresheners and multipurpose sprays—and found that they emitted more than 450 chemicals into the air, including a number of compounds linked to asthma, developmental and reproductive harm, or cancer. Use certified green products for all your cleaning. Just make sure that they will kill viruses and germs, and if not, use a natural disinfectant such as alcohol (with at least 70% alcohol content), hydrogen peroxide or vinegar in conjunction with your cleaner.

Your water supply is another concern. You might reassure yourself that buying bottled water is best, but the EWG conducted

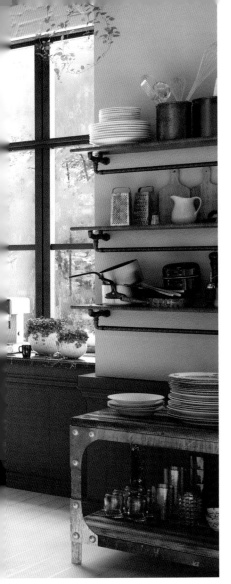

they use a lot of water during the filtration process. Simple carbon filters, such as Brita, that are used on your faucet or countertop are a great and cost-effective option."

Another potential source of toxins are the containers you use for food, especially plastic ones that come with takeout. Over the years the Food and Drug Administration has banned certain chemicals in plastics that are hormone disrupters, such as bisphenol A (BPA), for use in children's products such as infant bottles—but BPA affects adults as well. Avoid plastics marked with a 7, which may contain BPA, and never put plastics in the microwave or dishwasher, as BPAs can leach out when heated. Your best bet: Skip the plastics entirely and use glass containers. Also, when shopping, buy fresh or frozen fruits or veggies in lieu of canned foods, as many can linings may contain BPA.

a study on 10 different brands and found they contained 38 pollutants from disinfection by-products, industrial chemicals and bacteria, according to Young. That's because, unlike water utilities whose H2O is regularly tested, the bottled-water industry rarely reports any contamination. The solution: Use tap water, but filter it. "Reverse osmosis filters seem to be the most comprehensive filters," says Young. "The drawback is that

Bathroom

Use the same green cleaners here as in the kitchen. Avoid harsh toilet and tile cleaners, which are loaded with chemicals. When it comes to personal-care items—makeup, deodorant, shampoo and moisturizer—look for natural brands. And sorry fragrance lovers: Avoid scented items. "Anything with the word *fragrance* on the label may contain phthalates, which are hormone disrupters," says Young.

For your shower, look for a non-vinyl shower curtain. (Hint: Vinyl will have the number 3 printed on the recycling seal, or the letters PVC.) Buy one made of cotton, nylon, polyester, or EVA or PEVA plastic. The VOCs in vinyl can become gaseous, triggering headaches and other woes. Also buy a filter for your showerhead, advises Young. "Many contaminants in tap water are aerosolized in hot water."

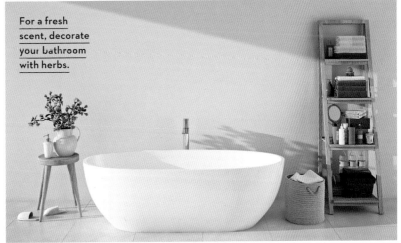

For a fresh scent, decorate your bathroom with herbs.

Rest & Reboot

ONE OF THE EASIEST (AND MOST ENJOYABLE!) WAYS TO DETOX IS THROUGH REGULAR, DEEP SLEEP—BUT MANY OF US STRUGGLE TO CATCH ENOUGH Z'S. HERE'S HOW TO FIX THAT.

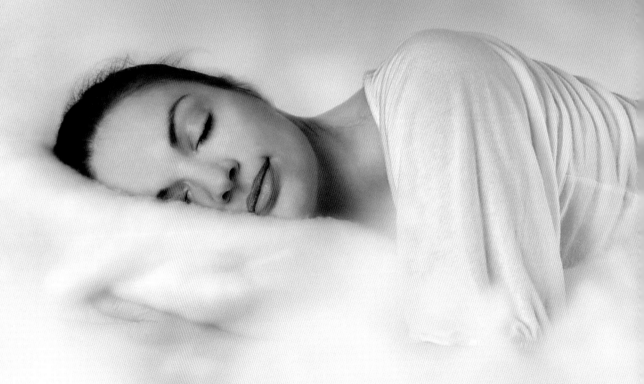

It's a no-brainer that *sleep* is good for you.

For proof, all you need to do is look back at the times when you've been sleep-deprived, whether you were caring for an infant or working into the wee hours. Perhaps you're among the one-third of Americans struggling with sleep issues right now. Lack of sleep leads to mental fogginess, weaker immune response (many college students get sick at the end of exam period) and weight gain.

According to the Centers for Disease Control and Prevention (CDC), routinely sleeping less than seven hours per night is linked to diabetes, high blood pressure, heart disease, stroke, obesity and depression. Hence, the CDC calls insufficient sleep a public health epidemic.

What you may not know, though, is that sleep also has a key function as a detoxifying agent—especially for your brain.

Better slumber is
more than a fantasy.

"Sleeping allows your brain to reorganize and recharge itself, as well as remove toxic waste by-products that have accumulated throughout the day," says Gavin Van De Walle, MS, RD, president of Dakota Dietitians. Adequate rest also has a powerful effect on your hormones, including some that control appetite and satiety, which helps explain why lack of sleep is so closely tied to obesity. Here's how sleep works—and how to get more of it.

Sleep for a Clear Head

A widely cited study in the journal *MEDtube Science*, titled "The Neuroprotective Aspects of Sleep," explains that in the normal like a plumbing system. It's a combination of the words *glia* and *lymphatic*: The lymphatic system is a network of tissues and organs that help rid the body of toxins and waste, and glial cells are the brain's helper cells, carrying nutrients to neurons, cleaning up dead nerve cells and other debris, and aiding communication between neurons.

The problem is that the brain can do only one task at a time, explain the authors, "whether it be clearing cellular waste products or processing sensory information, it cannot do both." Waste won't be cleared until your brain's neurons go to bed for the night. This is especially key because one form of waste that can pile up is a sticky, toxic

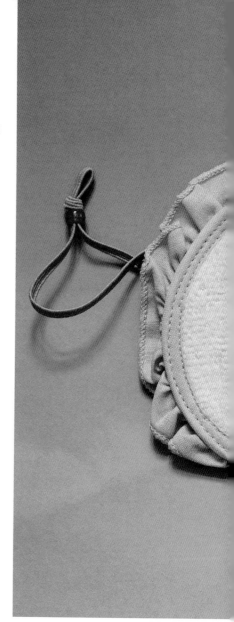

Solid rest is a *restoration* for your system.

course of cellular activity, the neurons in your brain produce waste by-products. An important role of sleep, the authors posit, is to "act like a garbage disposal for the brain," clearing out the debris so your brain can function normally the next day. It does that through a network called the glymphatic system, a waste clearance pathway that works protein called beta-amyloid, and one theory of Alzheimer's disease is that a buildup of beta-amyloid disrupts communication between brain cells. That helps explain the association that has been shown between long-term sleep problems and dementia.

Another important role of sleep in the brain is to help consolidate and store memories, says neuropsychiatrist Louann Brizendine, MD, author of *The Female Brain* and *The Male Brain*. During slow-wave (deep) sleep, your brain takes another look at memories that are in short-term storage in the hippocampus and decides which ones should go into long-term storage. "If you're short on slow-wave sleep, some memories can get left behind."

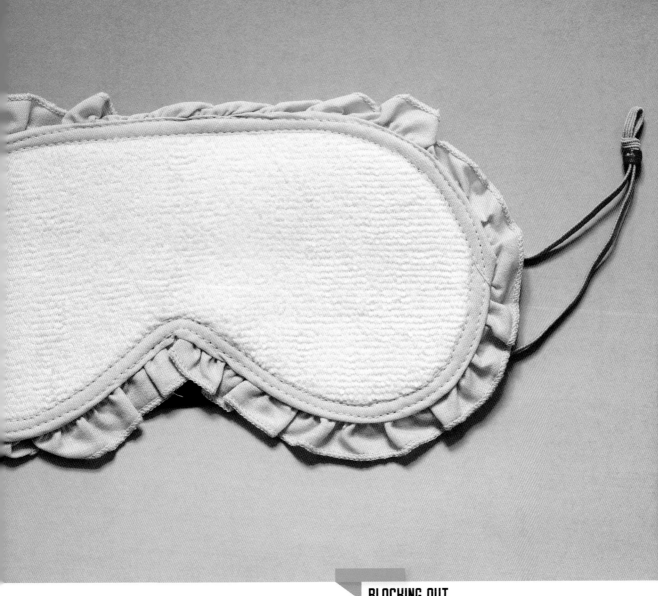

Sleep for Weight Loss

Research has repeatedly shown a strong association between sleep deprivation and weight gain, and there appear to be several mechanisms at work. One involves the hormones ghrelin (which increases appetite) and leptin (which reduces appetite). Normally, these hormones balance each other well, with leptin rising after you eat so you stay satiated for a few hours, and ghrelin kicking in when your body needs refueling. But getting less than the recommended seven to eight hours of solid rest throws both of them out of whack.

A study in the journal *Sleep* looked at two groups of young

BLOCKING OUT ANY AMBIENT LIGHT IS KEY.

adults, one of which slept fewer than five hours a night for four days straight, while the other slept normally during those nights. The sleep-deprived group showed overall higher levels of ghrelin and lower levels of leptin. Those hormones appeared to affect how they ate: The short sleepers snacked more, especially

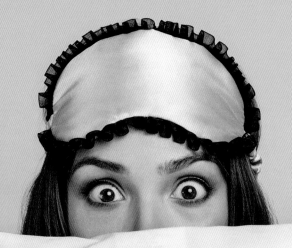

Don't go to
bed feeling
stressed.

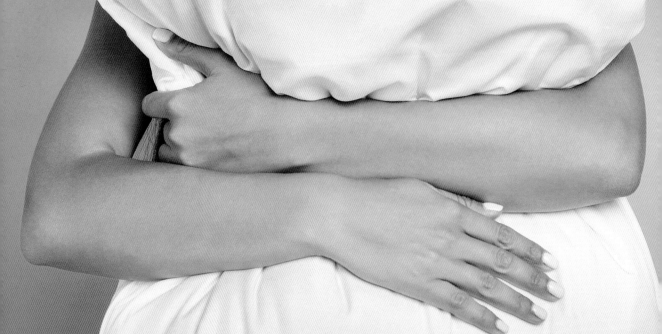

on foods that had more fat and protein, and the reward centers in their brains were also more susceptible to stimulation. This pattern suggests that sleep restriction may make the act of eating itself more satisfying.

A week of inadequate sleep (fewer than six hours a night) was also shown in one study to lead people to eat almost 700 calories more per day than those who slept at least seven hours. And in fact, as the amount of sleep reported by the average adult has declined over the past 40 years, the rate of obesity has soared. When your hormones are telling you to eat—and your brain is responding more strongly to the temptations of high-fat foods (i.e., junk food)—it's considerably more difficult to eat clean and control your weight.

Sleep Aids

No, not narcotics! These are some natural ways to reset your circadian rhythm and get the best rest:

Get Sunshine

Our bodies are set up to respond to day and night appropriately, but we throw things out of alignment with our modern lifestyle. Exposing yourself to sunshine every day helps teach your body when to be awake and alert, and when it's time for bed.

Reduce Blue-Light Exposure

The screens we look at all day emit a blue light that impacts our circadian rhythm, tricking it into thinking it's still daytime. Consider installing an app that blocks blue light on your smartphone, wearing glasses that block blue light, or just turning off the TV and other screens two hours before bedtime.

Cut Coffee—and Naps

There's a lot to love about coffee, but not after 3 p.m. Studies show caffeine can linger in your blood for six to eight hours, disrupting your evening wind down. Similarly with naps: A half-hour doze can refresh and revive, but anything longer confuses your internal clock.

Keep to Habits

Studies show that people with irregular sleeping patterns—for instance, staying up later and waking later on weekends—reported poor sleep more often. Your body is a creature of habit, so help it out by sticking to a routine.

Cool Your Bedroom

Snuggling in a cool room tells your body it's time to hibernate. Sleep experts suggest setting the thermostat between 65 and 69.

The Optimal Bedroom Setup

Equip your sleeping space to maximize your rest with these accessories:

BLACKOUT CURTAINS

These do a great job of making your room completely dark, even when it's still bright out or you live in an area with streetlights. Some even have designs such as a sheer print overlay that are both elegant and very effective.

SOUND MACHINE

City dwellers, listen up: Block out annoying noises (sirens, car alarms, loud conversations) with these machines, which can range from simple white noise players to elegant, pick-your-favorite-sound patterns.

SLEEP TRACKER

Many smartphones and smartwatches allow you to track your rest and even get a "sleep score" to clue you in on your heart rate, time asleep (including your time in light, deep and REM stages), restlessness and more.

SLEEP EYE MASK

For total coverage and comfort, go for silk—it's gentler on the skin than other fabrics and won't tug or create sleep lines and creases around your eyes. Or pick an aromatherapy version with a helpful sleep-inducing scent such as lavender.

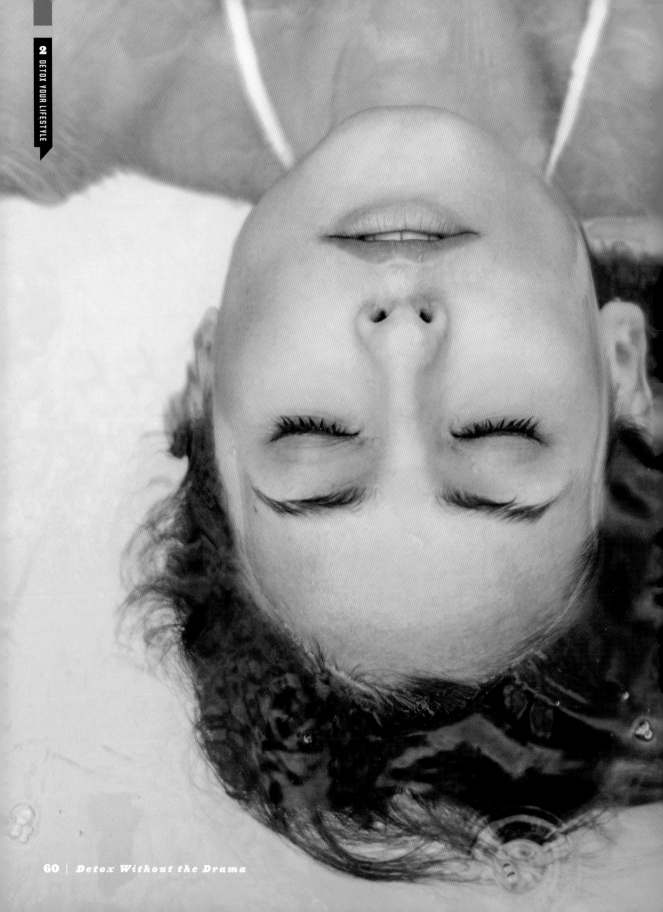

Taking the Waters

HYDRATING WITH PLAIN OLD H20 IS DETOXIFYING ALL BY ITSELF—
BUT YOU MAY WANT TO UP YOUR GAME WITH THESE STEPS.

For eons, water has been understood to be uniquely cleansing. From the ancient Romans through the 19th century, people who felt ill or suboptimal sought out hot springs and mineral springs for therapies. Those included both bathing (aka hydrotherapy) and drinking water from certain springs that were believed to be healing. In fact, the word *spa* is thought to have its origins in the letters—*s*, *p* and *a*—often scrawled as graffiti on the marble walls of ancient Roman public baths known as thermae. This may have been a coded message translated from the Latin, *salude per aqua*, which means "health [or healing] through water."

In the 18th and 19th centuries, spa towns such as Bath in England (which had ruins of Roman baths) and Karlsbad in Bohemia (now the Czech Republic) drew wealthy aristocrats to their resorts for the reputed healing effects of the local waters.

Now, with the advent of rigorous scientific studies, it appears that the ancients—and the Victorians—may have been onto something. Drinking water (and, some say, doing hydrotherapy as well) is one of the easiest, most basic ways to wash toxic or unhealthy substances

Fluids are like a *power wash* for your body.

out of your system. In part, that's because the movement of fluids through your body is one of its key detoxification pathways. The liver is our body's top detoxifying organ, but once it metabolizes the toxins they must be moved out of the body. That involves sweat as well as excretion through the digestive system—and all these systems function best when you're hydrating fully and often.

Here's how it works and how to stay in peak form.

Flushing It Out

On the most essential level, "water does much more than quench your thirst," says Gavin Van De Walle, MS, RD, owner of Dakota Dietitians. "It regulates your body temperature, lubricates joints, aids digestion and nutrient absorption, and detoxifies your body by removing waste products." Your body's cells must continuously be repaired to function optimally and break down nutrients for your body to use as energy, Van De Walle explains. "These processes release wastes, in the form of urea and carbon dioxide, that can

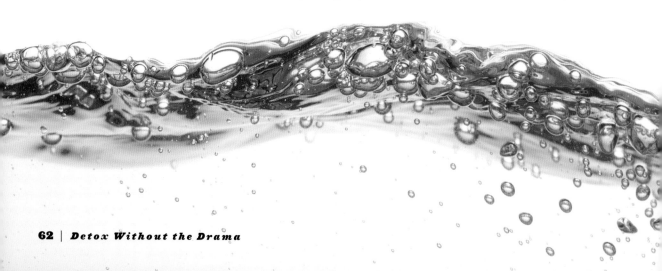

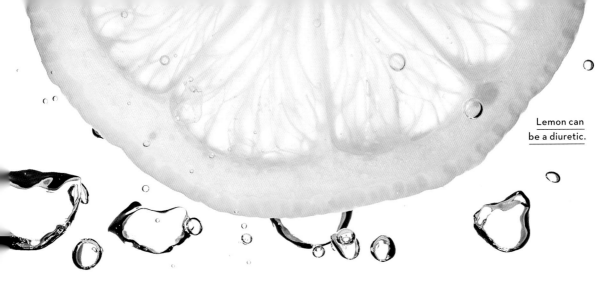

Lemon can be a diuretic.

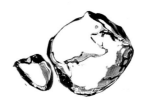

cause harm if allowed to build up in your blood." Water helps you wash those out of your body.

Taking in more water can also, ironically, help people whose systems retain too much water, says Van De Walle. "Consuming too much salt and not enough water can make your body retain excess fluid, causing bloating. That prompts your body to release an antidiuretic hormone that prevents you from urinating, and therefore detoxifying." The fix is simple: Drink more water. "That will reduce the secretion of the hormone and increase urination, eliminating more water and waste products."

Another way hydration helps you move toxins out? It's key to digestive health and maintaining regular bowel movements, another detoxification pathway. Studies in the *European Journal of Clinical Nutrition* and elsewhere have shown that dehydration can cause constipation. Your colon and large intestine are important organs in ridding your body of waste, and hydrating aids immensely in that process.

If one of your goals in detoxing is to drop a few pounds, drinking a lot of water is also your friend on that front. A study in the *Journal of Clinical Endocrinology & Metabolism* showed that drinking 17 ounces of water (about one-half liter) increased energy expenditure by 24% over the course of one hour after ingestion—a significant boost. Other research has shown that, whether due to metabolic reasons or a different mechanism, drinking water is associated with weight loss.

For instance, a study in the journal *Obesity* found that people on a low-calorie (weight-loss) diet who drank a half-liter of water before each meal lost

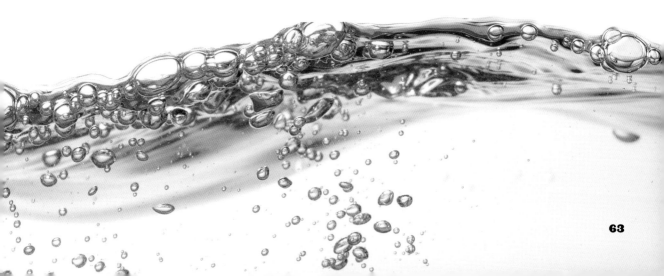

Water, Only Better

Detox water is a fancy name for a twist: H2O with pretty, and tasty, additions. It's easy to make, with a few caveats. For a hot drink, just pour boiling water over the ingredients and let steep for a few minutes. For cold drinks, add ingredients and put in the fridge for anywhere from one to 12 hours to allow the flavors to infuse (remove the ingredients after 12 hours to keep them from decomposing). In a hurry? Crush or bruise your fruit and herbs before using them to release the flavors more quickly.

Try these combos:

CUCUMBER AND MINT

LEMON AND GINGER

LEMON AND CAYENNE PEPPER

WATERMELON AND MINT

GRAPEFRUIT AND ROSEMARY

ORANGE AND LEMON

LEMON AND LIME

STRAWBERRY AND BASIL

APPLE AND CINNAMON

40% more weight over 12 weeks than those on the same diet who didn't drink water before their meals. The mechanisms of the weight loss have not yet been completely traced, but in addition to revving up your metabolic motor, it appears from research that drinking water is linked to appetite reduction.

Other Ways to Hydrate

If you've started to feel like you're floating away, consider taking in water through foods as well. Foods are a key hydrating source, which is why anyone doing an intermittent fast has to drink a lot of water to replace liquid they would normally take in from foods such as cucumber, lettuce and other produce.

The hydration you get from certain foods is different from the kind you get from water alone, according to Dana Cohen, MD, co-author of *Quench*. She describes a new "phase" of water called gel water, identified as H3O2, because it has extra atoms of both hydrogen and oxygen. "This is the phase that's found in our cells and also found in nature in plants," says Cohen. "Think of aloe and cactus, think of iceberg lettuce and chia seeds all loaded with gel water. By eating more plants, we are hydrating more efficiently than drinking more and more water." Gel water is absorbed more deeply into your muscles, cells and fascia, the connective tissue of your body, says Cohen. "Its absorptive qualities—picture the gel-like substance that forms around chia seeds when you soak them—help the body retain water."

That's not to say plain old water isn't useful as well, Cohen adds. Her prescription: First, front-load your water intake by drinking eight to 16 ounces first thing in the morning with a pinch of sea salt (for electrolytes) and a squeeze of lemon (for minerals). Then, drink a green smoothie each day—with added chia seeds—for a good dose of gel water.

Detox Water

There are various claims about so-called detox water, which is basically just water that's been infused with fruits, vegetables or herbs. Some sources tout weight loss, toxin removal, balancing the body's pH, digestive health, better energy and an immune boost. Other experts say many of the benefits are due to the water itself, rather than the ingredients. But there are a few pluses to fancying up your water. For one thing, you're likely to drink more water overall since it has a bit more flavor to it. And squeezing fresh lemon juice into your water gives you a hit of vitamin C, potassium, magnesium and copper, while helping you absorb more nutrients, such as iron and calcium, from the other foods you eat.

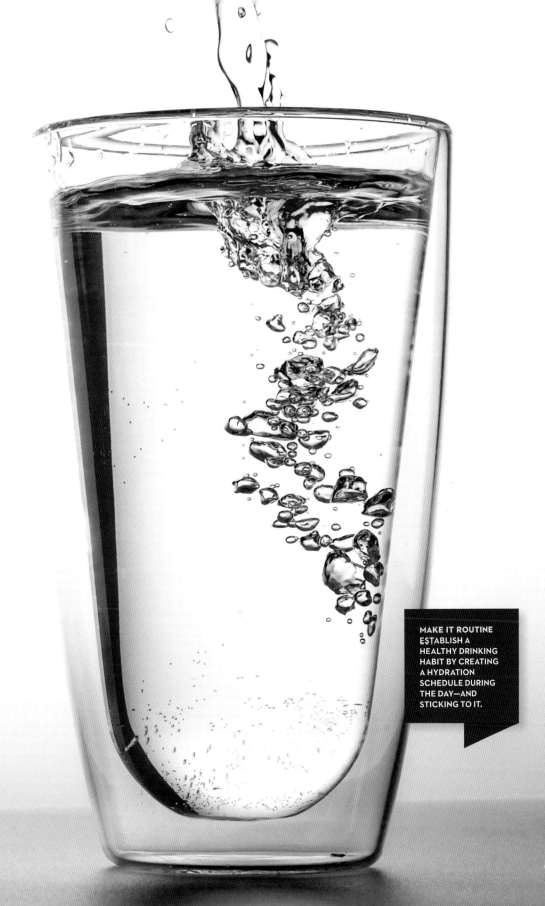

MAKE IT ROUTINE
ESTABLISH A
HEALTHY DRINKING
HABIT BY CREATING
A HYDRATION
SCHEDULE DURING
THE DAY—AND
STICKING TO IT.

Exercise
boosts mood
in just a few
minutes.

Working Out the Toxins

GETTING YOUR HEART AND BLOOD PUMPING HELPS MOVE THE BAD STUFF OUT, BUT THE CLEANSING ASPECTS OF VIGOROUS EXERCISE GO FAR DEEPER THAN SIMPLY BETTER CIRCULATION.

The health benefits of exercise are undisputed: a lower risk of heart disease and cancer, weight control and blood-sugar control, anti-aging effects, and many others. Now more and more research is suggesting that some of these life-extending benefits are directly related to the detoxing and cleansing aspect of exercise.

That shouldn't be too surprising when you consider how many of the pathways of detoxing are related to exercise. Your lungs, kidneys, circulation, digestive tract and lymph and immune systems are all key to detoxing, and they all come into play when you're active. Here's how it works—and how to work exercise into your detox plan.

All Systems Go

"Exercise accelerates the detoxification process," says internist Eva Cwynar, MD. First, she explains, by raising your heart rate, working out "pushes the blood to circulate more efficiently through the body, allowing nutrients to more easily reach all the organs and muscles." Second, and especially central to cleansing, Cwynar says, is the way exercise "helps lymph fluids circulate through the body, which removes toxins and other harmful materials." The lymphatic system is a network of tissues and organs that helps rid the body of toxins, waste and other unwanted materials (such as damaged or dying cells and proteins). It is also an important part of your immune system, helping to protect against infection and illness. It functions largely by transporting lymph, a fluid containing infection-fighting white cells, throughout the body.

"When you think of fluids in the body, you think of blood. But you have about five liters of blood in your body, and 15 liters of lymph," says Peter Bennett, ND, co-author of *7-Day Detox Miracle*. "A lot of toxins and metabolic by-products

that have been swept out of your cells, they're carried away by the lymphatic system." Just moving your body in any way boosts this process, says Bennett. "Your muscles contract, and that circulates the lymph."

Exercise also increases respiration—and the lungs are another essential part of your natural detoxing system. When you breathe deeply during exercise it helps empty your lungs of carbon dioxide and other toxins and bring in more oxygen and nourishment to all your cells.

exercise and a decrease in inflammation, which is one of the main targets of a detox. A paper published in the *Journal of Applied Physiology* found that a group of 75-year-old men who were lifelong aerobic exercisers had inflammation profiles much closer to those of 25-year-old regular exercisers than to those of their healthy 75-year-old peers who were sedentary.

Another study, in the journal *Brain, Behavior, and Immunity*, found that just 20 minutes of walking on a treadmill produced

Regular exercise helps *fight* inflammation.

Physical activity plays a role in digestion as well: It has been shown to aid healthy flora in the microbiome, which strengthens your gut walls and enables your body to more efficiently remove toxins through the large intestine.

Special Benefits

Moving your body does more than just stimulate and intensify your body's natural detoxification pathways, however. Recent research is showing changes at the cellular level that promote cleansing. Several studies have found a direct link between

an anti-inflammatory cellular response, reducing the activity of cells called cytokines that can promote inflammation. Other research has shown that when you do any kind of exercise, your muscle cells release a small protein called interleukin-6 (IL-6), which plays an important role in fighting inflammation; a 30-minute workout will increase IL-6 fivefold. Another protein that goes up with exercise, interleukin-15 (IL-15), helps to protect against abdominal fat buildup. Since fat around the middle is itself thought to promote inflammation (partly by releasing toxins into nearby organs), the increase in IL-15 may act to lower overall inflammation levels.

And if you're hoping that your detox will also help lower your stress levels—well, exercise does that, too. It has been thought that the mental benefits of exercise are related to the release of endorphins, but that's not all.

Researchers at Sweden's Karolinska Institutet found that exercise raises levels of a substance in the muscles that may protect the brain from stress-induced depression. "We found that well-trained muscles produce an enzyme that purges the body of harmful substances" known to accumulate during stress, says study co-author Jorge Ruas. "Skeletal muscle appears to have a detoxification effect that, when activated, can protect the brain from depression and related mental illness."

Working It In

So what to do, and how much, as part of your detox? "A little aerobic exercise every day is good for everyone, but especially during detoxification," says Bennett. "That can be bicycling, jogging, swimming, brisk walking—anything that raises your heart rate for 20 minutes, ideally at least three times a week. Jumping rope is particularly

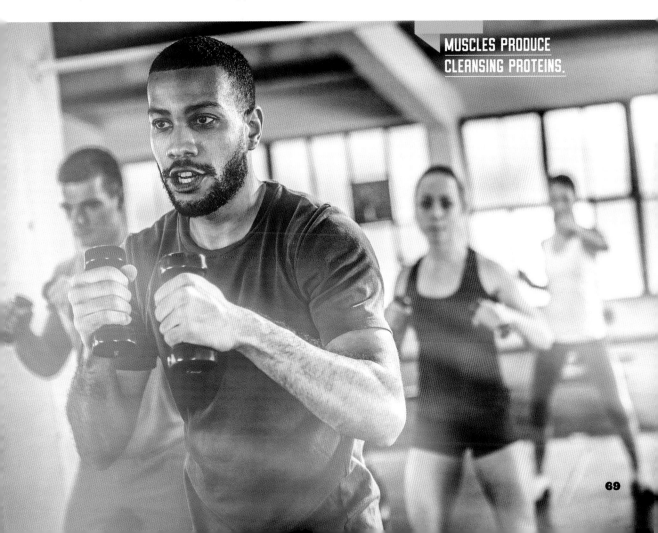

MUSCLES PRODUCE CLEANSING PROTEINS.

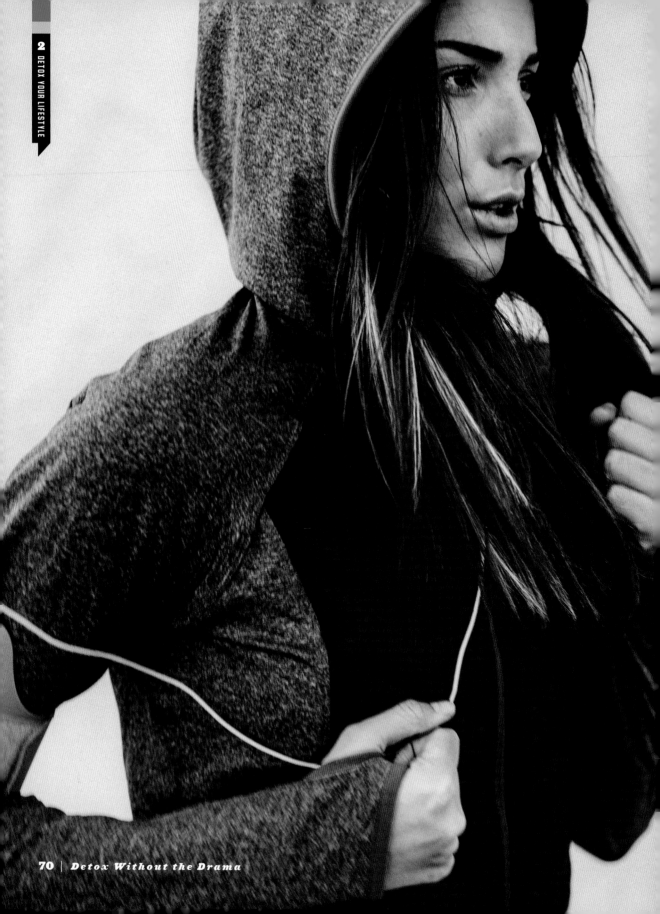

useful, Bennett says. "It's a good workout that increases aerobic capacity, timing and coordination. It's excellent for the calves, hips, thighs and abdominal muscles."

The activity doesn't need to be superintense—some doctors even advise keeping to moderate exercise during a detox, when you're likely restricting sources of quick energy like simple carbs. The point isn't to push yourself to the max, but simply to get things moving. Eastern forms of movement such as yoga and qigong are also good for cleansing not only your body but also your mind, and both include exercises specifically to spur detoxing.

Weight lifting, or strength training, is an excellent choice as well. To avoid injury, don't start too heavy, and build up your strength as you go. Aim to do some form of full-body strength training 2-3 days a week. Working with weights builds muscle, helps you burn more fat on a regular basis, and also releases helpful proteins and hormones. Strength training has been shown to increase levels of human growth hormone (HGH), which helps cells rejuvenate, and an anti-aging protein called s-Klotho, which inhibits cell aging and preserves stem cells. Talk about a fountain of youth!

Sweat It Out!

Welcome that workout glow—it's helping to cleanse your system.

Getting your sweat on can be a helpful element in your detox. A study in the *Journal of Environmental and Public Health* found that heavy metals can be excreted in sweat, including arsenic, cadmium, lead and mercury. "Athletes have been shown to have lower levels of toxins, because they sweat more," says Peter Bennett, ND; his *7-Day Detox Miracle* plan includes regular sauna sessions.

"The sweat glands are a major thoroughfare for the elimination of toxins," Bennett says. "Fluids in the blood and lymph are 'sacrificed' to manufacture sweat. When we sweat, some of the poisons these fluids contain are excreted through the skin. Your skin acts like a second kidney." Your body also stores many toxins in fatty tissue, Bennett adds, and "sweating reduces fat stores, releasing these

poisons for excretion." In traditional rituals—including Ayurveda and Native American—sweating plays an integral role in detoxing.

You must drink a lot of water, though. While sweating intensely, a person can lose as many as three liters of fluid in an hour, says Bennett, so drink up constantly. The fluid intake also speeds your detox by helping your kidneys flush out toxins through excretion.

Your skin, another element in your natural detox system, also benefits from a good sweat. It unclogs pores, letting toxins out, and the water, salt and minerals in sweat hydrate and exfoliate the skin. Sweat also rids the skin of dirt, bacteria and oils, and contains an antimicrobial peptide called dermcidin, which helps fight off germs. After a sweat, take a cool shower to help close your pores.

The Yoga Cleanse

IT'S NOT NECESSARILY HEART POUNDING OR SWEATY,
BUT THE AGE-OLD PRACTICE PLAYS A UNIQUE ROLE IN DETOXING
AND HEALING THE BODY.

When you think of supporting gut health—a critical element in the detoxing process—yoga may not be the first thing that comes to mind. After all, yoga doesn't entail eating! But the most powerful healing processes are integrative, involving nourishing the body in ways that go beyond food: using your muscles, circulation and lymphatic system to carry out toxins and cleanse the body. A yoga practice can help optimize functioning of the intestines, stimulate certain key organs involved in cleansing (such as the liver and pancreas) and improve circulation.

Studies have also shown that practicing yoga can decrease the secretion of cortisol, the primary stress hormone that also influences levels of serotonin, the neurotransmitter often associated with depression. This change in cortisol levels reduces feelings of stress, depression, anxiety and fatigue. And intriguingly, a study of 131 people who did yoga sessions regularly for 10 weeks showed lower levels of inflammatory markers, a key target of detox programs. Yet another cleansing benefit: Research has found that regular yoga practitioners are able to fall asleep faster, sleep longer and feel more well rested in the morning—and sleep is one of nature's best cleansers. **Try the following five poses to get the best detoxing benefits:**

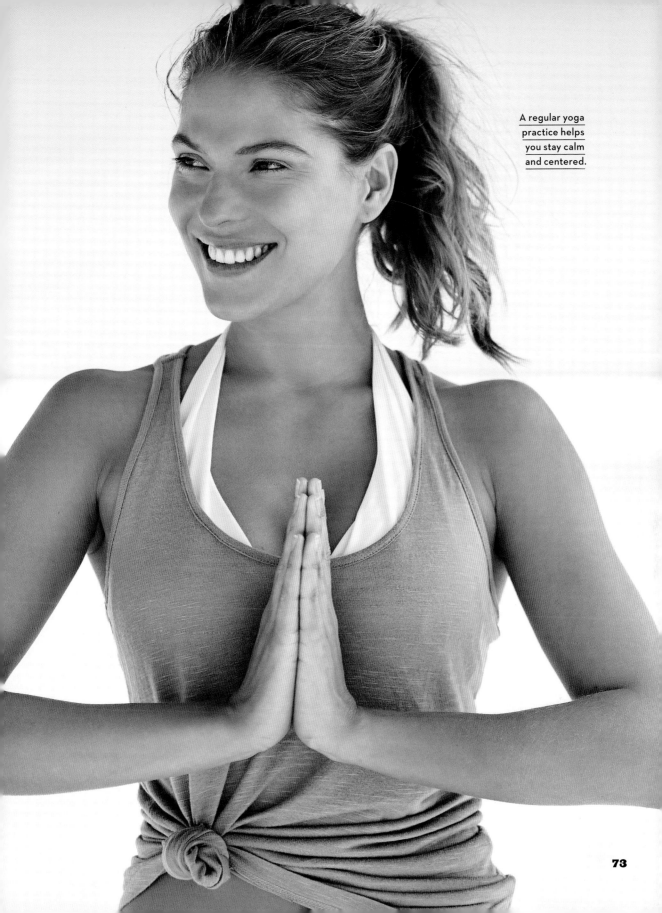

A regular yoga practice helps you stay calm and centered.

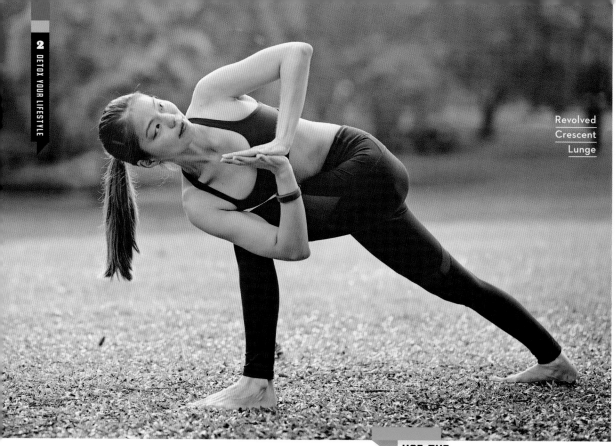

Revolved
Crescent
Lunge

**USE THE
BREATH TO
DETOXIFY.**

1 Revolved Crescent Lunge

A majority of the twist postures in yoga aid digestion and gut health. This is because you're applying pressure to the areas associated with the digestive system, in order to release toxins. Think of it as giving your internal organs a massage. Revolved Crescent Lunge is great for helping relieve constipation, bloating and other digestive discomfort. Undigested foods, fluids and other toxins can get stuck in the intestinal tract, which is why twists are so useful for stimulating the gut and eliminating waste.

How to Do It Start from a High Lunge position, where your front (left) knee is stacked over your left ankle, and the right leg is extended long behind the body, with the ball of the foot tracking over the heel. From here, bring your hands to prayer position at heart center and begin to twist from the torso toward the left, hooking your right elbow to the outside of the left knee, extending your left elbow to the sky. The crown of the head is reaching toward the front, with a long line of energy extending from the crown out through the heel of the back foot. With every inhale, elongate the spine, and with every exhale, use the elbow as leverage to twist deeper, opening up the chest. Be mindful in this pose that the back (right) leg does not collapse; rather, imagine lifting through the thigh in order to maintain integrity.

Feel free to drop to the back knee for a modification and oftentimes a deeper twist, "rinsing" out the internal organs. Then switch sides, lunging forward with your right leg and extending the left leg back. Repeat four times.

2 Prayer Twist

This pose works similarly to the Revolved Crescent Lunge. In twists, the blood supply to the organs is constricted, so when you release from the pose, fresh blood is introduced to help remove waste and impurities from the cells. Twists also compress the colon, helping to stimulate regular bowel movements and adding further support to the body's own detoxification pathways. **How to Do It** Come into Chair Pose: Bring both feet together with a slight separation in the heels, knees touching, shifting the weight back into the heels and bending the knees about 90 degrees (just like a squat). From here, in one fluid motion, extend both arms over the head and bring your palms together, hands at heart center. Begin to slowly transition toward twisting to the right side by placing the left elbow outside the right knee, right elbow extending toward the sky. Make sure the knees are still in alignment by shifting the left

Use caution with inversions such as *Legs Up the Wall* if you have neck or back issues.

hip back. Open the chest toward the side as you use the left elbow as leverage to get a little deeper into the twist. Stay here for three to five breaths, finding length

through the torso and crown of the head on the inhale and twisting deeper on each exhale. Release the twist and return to chair pose, extending the arms high, and then repeat the same motion on the opposite side. Release the posture by coming into a Forward Fold, bending the knees so that the belly rests on the thighs and the head and arms hang down heavy toward the mat. Repeat four times.

3 Bow Pose
This pose supports gut health by applying gentle pressure to the belly, stimulating the digestive system. Rocking forward and backward on your abdomen to the rhythm of your inhales and exhales offers a gentle massage to the internal

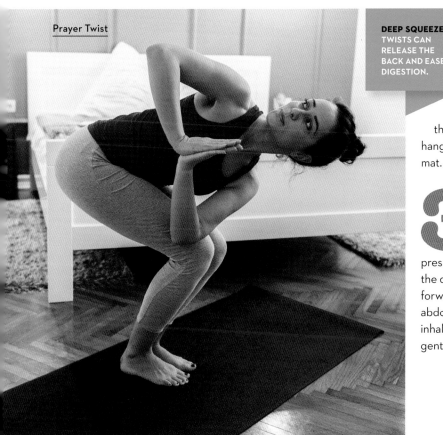

Prayer Twist

DEEP SQUEEZE TWISTS CAN RELEASE THE BACK AND EASE DIGESTION.

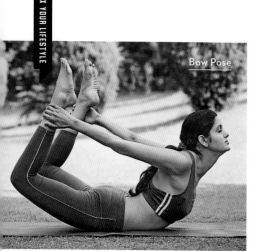

Bow Pose

4 Sun Salutation

In Hindu theory, digestion occurs through producing heat, and food is burned to create energy. One of the best ways to produce heat is by doing Sun Salutation. They often begin a yoga class, warming up your body before doing more complex poses. Sun Salutation detoxifies through inhalation and exhalation, oxygenating the blood and eliminating carbon dioxide. **How to Do It** Start in Mountain Pose, finding a steady foundation, and bring hands to heart center. On your next inhale, reach arms high and exhale your hands through heart center into a forward fold, hinging at the hips and keeping a flat back. On the next inhale, bend further and bring hands toward the floor in a half lift, keeping a long, straight spine; you may need to micro-bend at the knees. Exhale, plant your hands, and flow through your vinyasa,

starting with Low Plank (body straight, parallel to the floor, arms bent, elbows grazing the sides of the ribs). Inhale into Upward-Facing Dog, arching your back and opening your chest; then lead with the low belly pressing back to Downward-Facing Dog. Complete this sequence three to five times, moving at the pace of your inhales and exhales.

5 Legs Up the Wall

This is an inversion, with the head below the heart, which improves circulation by reversing blood flow. This also aids digestion by sending blood to the gut, and helps restore you after a day spent on your feet. It drains the legs of metabolic waste and helps clear the lymphatic system. **How to Do It** Have a folded blanket or towel, block or small pillow handy for support under the low back/sacrum. Find a

organs, oxygenating them by increasing blood flow. This helps relieve constipation or other gut-health issues, aiding in elimination and removing waste and toxins. **How to Do It** Lie flat on your stomach with your hands extended along your sides, palms facing down. Slowly begin to grab hold of your right foot or ankle with your right hand and then your left foot or ankle with your left hand. Keeping your thighs on the ground and your gaze facing down toward the mat, begin to lift your chest on an inhale by kicking your feet upward into your hands. Lift your gaze forward, extending your heart to the front. If you can, slowly lift your thighs off the ground, pressing your heart farther toward the front and opening your chest. Deepen your inhales and exhales enough so that it causes you to roll forward and backward on your abdomen. Stay here for three to five deep breaths, then release to the mat. Repeat four times.

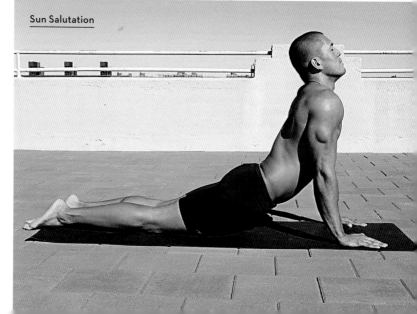

Sun Salutation

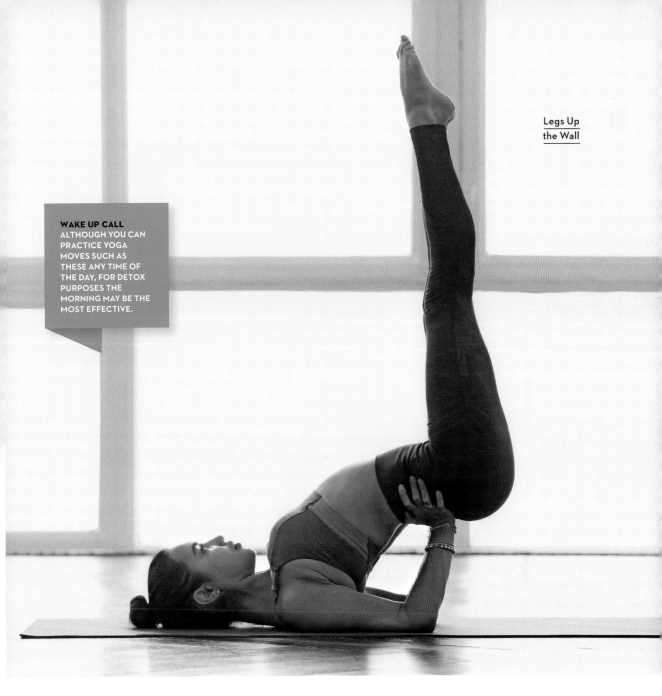

Legs Up
the Wall

WAKE UP CALL
ALTHOUGH YOU CAN
PRACTICE YOGA
MOVES SUCH AS
THESE ANY TIME OF
THE DAY, FOR DETOX
PURPOSES THE
MORNING MAY BE THE
MOST EFFECTIVE.

comfortable seat facing a wall (or you can do the pose without one if you are more advanced), with knees bent so that the tips of your toes touch the wall. Slowly recline to your back, keeping knees bent. Once reclined, start walking your feet up the wall one inch at a time. Make micro-movements to "inchworm" your body closer to the wall, so your legs are parallel resting against the wall. Reach for your support (pillow, block, etc.) and place it under your sacrum (if you are advanced, use your hands for support). Keep legs engaged, firm but not stiff; you can bend your knees slightly or separate feet hip-width distance. Find what's comfortable and stay five to 10 minutes, softening areas where you may be holding tension. To come out, slowly bend the knees and release the feet to the ground.

Deep breathing is one of the best ways to reduce stress right when you're feeling it the most.

Fresh Breath

YOU DO IT THOUSANDS OF TIMES A DAY WITHOUT EVEN THINKING ABOUT IT, BUT BEING MINDFUL ABOUT EACH INHALE AND EXHALE CAN HELP REDUCE STRESS, BOOST ENERGY, REDUCE TOXINS AND EVEN MAKE YOU FEEL HAPPIER.

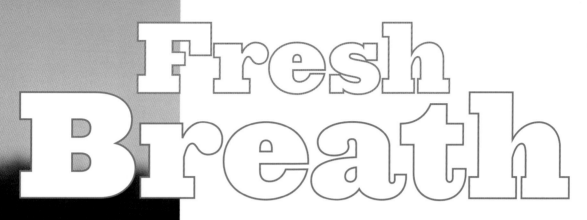

Breathing isn't something you tend to think about very much. Unless you're deliberately holding it (trying to cure hiccups) or struggling to maintain it (hiking at elevation), breathing just comes naturally.

But this most basic function plays a big part in your health. With every inhalation, you draw in oxygen to nourish the cells; with every exhale, you release carbon dioxide and other waste products.

And that's not all: Your breath plays a fundamental role in the relaxation response—your ability to fight stress in the moment. The more you can control your breathing, the faster you can regain a sense of calm.

"When you are stressed, the sympathetic branch of the autonomic nervous system [the subconscious part of the nervous system that regulates functions such as heart rate and digestion, breathing, metabolism and much more] becomes activated, signalling the 'fight-or-flight' response," explains Patricia Gerbarg, MD, an assistant clinical professor of psychiatry at New York Medical College. You know this one—your heart speeds up, your stomach starts to churn, your palms may sweat. When you're constantly stressed or worried, this response can get overloaded, contributing to many of the major diseases of aging. Deep breathing stimulates the parasympathetic nervous system, helping you regain your composure.

Slowing Down

Of all the autonomic functions in the body, the only one you can really voluntarily control is your breathing. After all, you can't make your heart rate speed up or your digestion slow down just by thinking about it. But by consciously changing how you breathe—the rate, depth and pattern—you can change the messages your body sends to your brain.

"There are billions of receptors throughout your lungs, diaphragm and chest walls, so a huge amount of information is picked up every time you breathe in and out," says Gerbarg. All of these receptors send signals throughout the nervous system, but especially through the vagus nerve, which leads straight to the brain. "Since respiration is so critical to our survival, the brain listens very closely to these signals," she adds. Having this ability to control your breath is crucial. Breathing can help to alleviate some of the negative feelings (anxiety, depression, fear) and bring out more positive ones (love, compassion) simply by calming down the fight-or-flight response and helping your body regain a sense of control.

Gerbarg recommends practicing what's known as coherent breathing, which involves taking five or six slow and steady breaths per minute. "We've found that breathing more rapidly, say seven to eight breaths a minute, can be calming but it's not as relaxing. And taking only three to four breaths a minute can put you in an almost meditative state, but you're not quite as alert. Five to six breaths a minute is the sweet spot."

While Gerbarg helps to teach workshops that focus on how to master coherent breathing (see her website, breath-body-mind .com), you can also try practicing on your own. Focus on breathing in fully for a count of five and exhaling fully for a count of five. Practice doing this for about 10 minutes at a time, ideally twice a day, says Gerbarg, and you'll soon be able to call on this as a tool whenever your stress levels start to rise. Over time, your breath rate

> **5 TO 6**
> THE NUMBER OF SLOW BREATHS TO TAKE IN ONE MINUTE TO FIGHT STRESS. THAT'S ABOUT FIVE SECONDS EACH FOR INHALING AND EXHALING.

Deep breaths give tissues *more oxygen.*

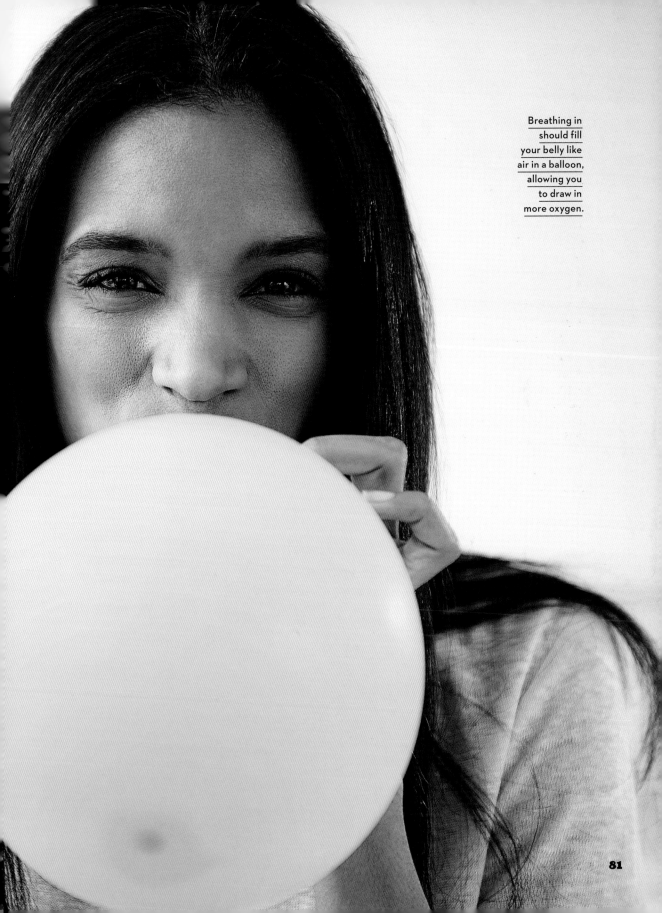

Breathing in
should fill
your belly like
air in a balloon,
allowing you
to draw in
more oxygen.

may naturally come down, allowing you to draw in more oxygen. (That's a bonus for athletes who take part in endurance sports such as running, since the more oxygen you draw in, the more efficient you become and the less energy you need to expend.)

Body Breathe

Some therapists think we need to go beyond deep-breathing techniques to change the way we actually breathe. "So many of us breathe from the upper chest and shoulders, rather than from the diaphragm," notes Belisa Vranich,

PhD, a clinical psychologist and author of *Breathe*. Rather than breathing vertically, as Vranich calls it, we need to focus on expanding and softening the belly. "Ask a 5-year-old to inhale, and he will usually puff out his belly without thinking about it," says Vranich. "By the time we're adults, many of us take this breathing mostly into our chest."

Think of it this way: Ideally, you should expand and soften as you inhale, like a balloon that's expanding. Then, as you let the air out, focus on tightening your midsection. Many of us do the

Techniques to Try

There's no shortage of deep-breathing exercises that can play a role in the detox process by lowering levels of stress hormones. Consider these tried-and-true methods to increase the relaxation response and calm you down whenever you feel stressed.

ALTERNATE NOSTRIL BREATHING
Boost energy and focus by breathing through one nostril at a time.
1 Cover right nostril with right thumb.
2 Slowly inhale through left nostril.
3 Cover your left nostril with your ring finger so both sides are closed for a moment.
4 Uncover your right nostril and slowly breathe out.
5 Slowly inhale through your right nostril.

6 Cover your right nostril so both sides are closed for a moment.
7 Uncover your left nostril and slowly breathe out.
8 Repeat these steps five times.

ROLL BREATHING
Expand lung capacity with deep belly breaths.
1 Lie on your back with knees bent, left hand on belly and right hand on chest.
2 Take a deep breath through your nose

and fill your lower lungs so that only your belly (not your chest) rises when you inhale.
3 Breathe out slowly through your mouth.
4 Repeat 10 times.
5 Continue breathing in through your nose and out through your mouth; make a soft whooshing sound as you exhale.
6 When you inhale, fill your belly with air before your upper chest; your chest should rise slightly as your belly falls.

7 Continue this pattern for three to five minutes.

4-7-8 BREATHING
Induce natural relaxation by making exhalations twice as long as inhalations:
1 Close your mouth and inhale through your nose. Silently count to four.
2 Hold for a count of seven.
3 Exhale through your mouth as you silently count to eight.
4 Repeat these steps at least three times.

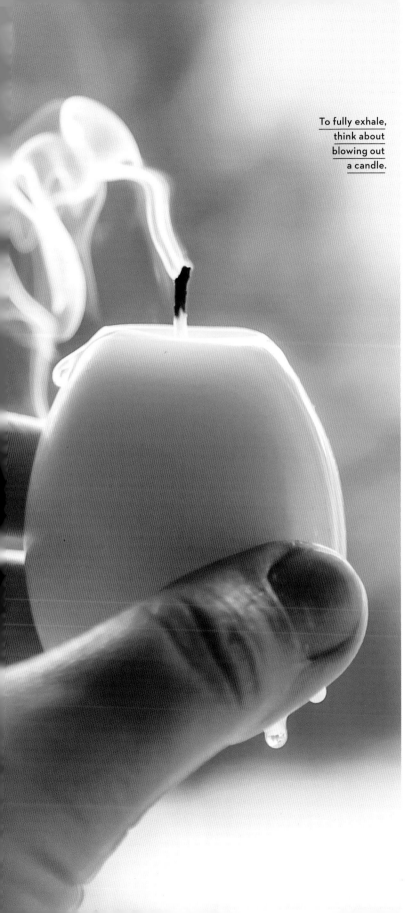

To fully exhale, think about blowing out a candle.

opposite—pulling the gut in as we inhale, like trying to zip up a tight pair of pants. "The problem is, you'll take in significantly less air this way," explains Vranich. Another common issue is holding your breath for no reason. There are also overbreathers (breathing at a high rate) and "no-halers," says Vranich, who don't take significant inhalations or exhalations, but rather "hover" with a shallow breath rate. All of these methods cut down the amount of oxygen your body takes in and how much carbon dioxide you breathe out.

Poor posture also comes into play. "So many of us sit for a huge percentage of the day—up to 16 hours—and when you sit, you simply don't breathe as well," notes Vranich. "That's a long time for lower levels of oxygen to be passing through your body."

Instead, think about engaging your diaphragm with every breath you take. "One breath using your diaphragm is worth four to six breaths coming from the top part of your body," she says. Psychologically, lower-body breathing is also more calming, while upper-body breaths can put you in a more stressed-out state. That, in turn, can affect everything from sleep patterns to digestion.

Ready to give it a go? See "Techniques to Try," on opposite page—these three methods can help you feel calmer, more energized and rejuvenated, all in a matter of minutes.

Clear Your Mind, Clear Your Body

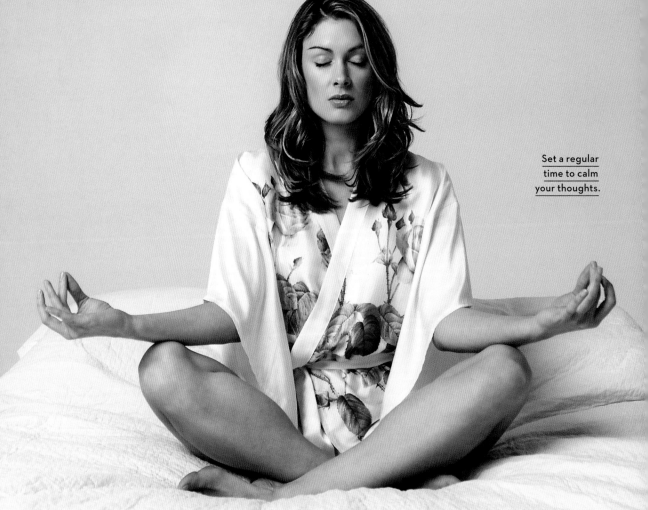

Set a regular time to calm your thoughts.

STRESS IS JUST AS DESTRUCTIVE TO YOUR SYSTEM AS MORE EASILY IDENTIFIED TOXINS—WHICH IS WHY A MEDITATION PRACTICE SHOULD BE PART OF ANY CLEANSE.

Meditation may not involve drinking celery juice or cutting out sugar, but it does play a surprisingly powerful role in a detoxing regimen. While it's been practiced in some cultures for thousands of years, it's only more recently that science has realized its potency, not only for psychological balance but also for physical health.

Recent evidence includes a study in the journal *Molecular Psychiatry*, which showed that feeling stress actively counteracted the effects of a healthy diet (lesson learned: Diet alone is only one part of optimal health). And one of the first effects of meditation is lower stress levels. Research into meditation and mindfulness in general has exploded to such a degree that each year several thousand studies are published on the topic.

Many of these studies are showing that if the goal of your cleanse is to improve your overall health, strengthen your immune response and clear your system of toxins, then bringing your brain into the equation is an important tool in your toolbox. Stress is a key player because it is a destructive force throughout your body. It's not just a matter of

feeling anxious; chronic stress is a major contributor to inflammation, prompting the release of stress hormones such as cortisol and adrenaline. "In large amounts, these hormones create toxins and slow down detoxification enzymes in the liver," says Linda Page, ND, PhD, author of *Healthy Healing*. "Yoga, qigong and meditation are simple and effective ways to relieve stress by resetting your physical and mental reactions to the inevitable stress life brings."

The Toll of Stress

Our bodies are intelligently designed to handle stress in moderate amounts, like the intermittent pressure to meet a deadline at work or the occasional overscheduled calendar. But the body is not equipped to handle chronic stress, the type that inflicts prolonged periods of tension in which you feel you have little control. Stress hormones are useful in the short term, helping you enter fight-or-flight mode, speeding up your heartbeat and pumping blood to critical areas of the body such as the muscles and heart. Once the stress subsides, the body responds by activating its rest-and-recovery system, maintaining homeostasis within the body. But when stress is

chronic, the body lives in an eternal state of inflammation, which has been linked to many health conditions, including hormone imbalance, heart conditions and digestive disorders.

That last item is so important, because the gut plays a significant role in optimal health. Nearly the entire immune system depends on the collection of healthy bacteria and fungi living within the large intestine, and undigested foods can be traced back to debilitating and toxifying conditions like leaky gut (which allows toxins to seep into the bloodstream) and dysbiosis (overgrowth of pathogens in the gut). During times of increased stress, blood is pumped toward critical areas of the body such as the heart, taking away from other areas such as the gut, ultimately impairing digestion. At the same time, chronic stress makes the heart pump faster, while blood vessels constrict to send oxygen toward the muscles as part of the fight-or-flight system, ultimately raising blood pressure. This is an added concern for those with preexisting heart conditions, and it also increases the risk for heart attack or stroke.

Although some level of stress is inevitable, we can mitigate

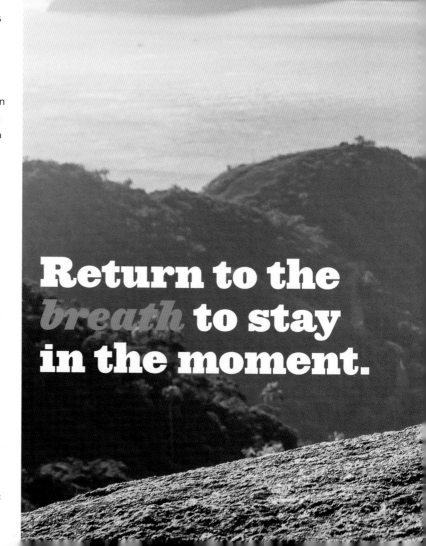

its negative impact by implementing coping mechanisms that help cleanse the mind of accumulated stressors. Meditation is one of those mechanisms, helping to detox from mental toxins—not to mention improving sleep patterns and lowering blood pressure. "Meditation is exercise for the mind," says Greg Reicks, DO, a family practitioner and yoga studio owner in Grand Junction, Colorado. "And we need to think about it as a means of preventive medicine, too." Reicks recommends meditation for his patients, in conjunction with other therapies, to reduce stress hormones. He says he even sees improvement in his patients with chronic pain when they try a routine meditation practice.

Getting Started

One major advantage of meditation is that it can be done anytime, anywhere, and does not require prior experience, gym membership, fancy props or special clothing. It's a process of linking thoughts and breath, in which you begin to control the stressors in your life rather than feeling engulfed by them.

The key to a successful and sustainable meditation practice is finding a technique that feels most comfortable for you. There are many ways to meditate—even walking in nature can be

GUT REACTION
THE BODY MUST BE IN A PARASYMPATHETIC STATE—CALM, COMPOSED AND RESTING—IN ORDER TO PROPERLY DIGEST FOOD.

Return to the *breath* to stay in the moment.

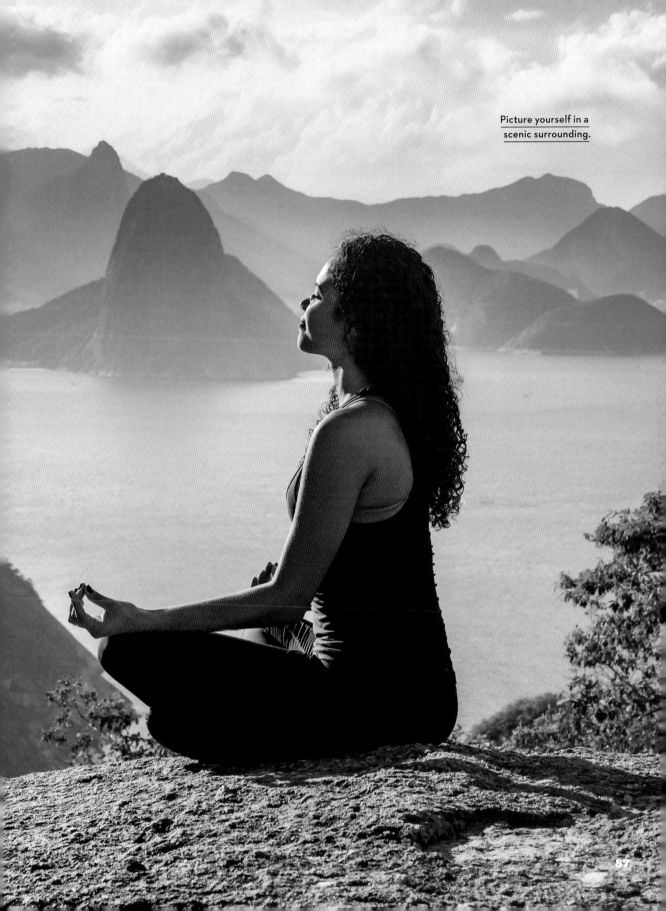

Picture yourself in a scenic surrounding.

Chronic stress
can take a toll
unless you
learn to cope.

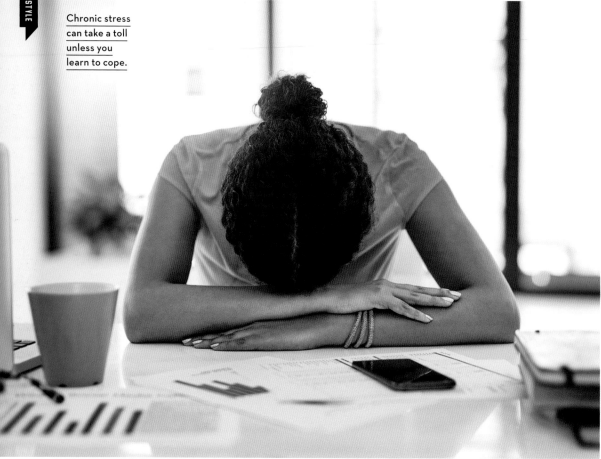

considered a form of meditation—but determining the practice that best fits you will help ensure that you can stick with it long term. "People have a hard time tuning out," Reicks says, "so I recommend that you think about meditation differently and start small. It could be as simple, at the beginning, as being aware of your inhales and exhales for 15 seconds." It's also important to choose a regular time for your meditation, and planning to incorporate at least a few sessions a week. For instance, perhaps you can take a few minutes before bed, sitting quietly and focusing on breath work, or pause for a mindfulness session during your lunch hour.

Stress may be unavoidable, but you can alleviate some of its side effects by harnessing your mind's own cleansing powers. After a few weeks, you'll find its effects will start impacting your everyday life: When you hit a rough patch, you'll take a cleansing breath and feel your heartbeat stabilize and your stomach unclench. Here are three methods to try as you look for the right fit.

Guided Meditation

This type of meditation evokes the senses by forming mental images that soothe and relax the body and mind. The easiest way to get started with a guided meditation is to use an app or podcast to lead you along. Some good options include the

Do a Device Detox

Another way to clear your head and promote calm:
Step away from the screen(s). Here's how.

Everywhere you look, people are bent over their smartphones, distracting themselves, multitasking—and inducing anxiety. It's almost the anti-meditation: Rather than emptying your mind, you're filling it with all kinds of detritus. And numerous studies show that frequent use of tech and phones, especially for social media such as Instagram and Snapchat, can increase depression, feelings of isolation and loneliness, and lower self-esteem. While it may seem extreme to call overuse of connective technology addictive, it does have elements of addiction, says David Greenfield, PhD, MS, assistant clinical professor of psychiatry at the University of Connecticut School of Medicine and founder of the Center for Internet and Technology Addiction. Pleasurable behaviors can be addictive, Greenfield says, because they induce a rush of the neurotransmitter dopamine, the "feel-good" chemical that interacts with the brain's reward centers, and can leave you wanting more. "In general, I would not say it's a life-threatening illness. It's a life-decreasing illness. It makes people unhealthier. It reduces people's ability to react in real time." Amp up the benefits of meditation by taking these steps.

1 START SLOW

Try a mini digital detox first: Turn off your phone for 15 minutes, work up to 30 minutes, and aim for a half or full day off the grid. This is especially key if you're a social media player, says Greenfield. "There's this idea that if others don't know you're doing something, it has no value. When you become an observer of the experience, rather than an experiencer of the experience, you're not really present." It's tough at first (Greenfield's research found that 50% of people felt withdrawal when they accidentally left their phones behind), but it gets easier, and more fulfilling, with practice.

2 USE APPS

It sounds counterintuitive—use my phone to stop using my phone?—but there are some great apps that can help you control your time online. One is Checky, which tells you how often you check your phone. "Most people are flabbergasted when they see they're checking it 300 times a day," says Greenfield. The Off the Grid app lets you set up device-free time in advance; it locks your phone down, but allows custom settings for important messages or calls.

3 CHANGE YOUR SETTINGS

In particular, turn off notifications. You don't need to get each news alert, sports score or friend's Insta-brag in real time.

4 PRACTICE TECH HYGIENE

Turn off your phone and put it away at meals. "The smartphone conveys to everyone you're with that you're not really psychologically there," Greenfield says. Carry a magazine or book (like this one!) with you instead of your phone; it focuses you on one thing at a time. Bring a pen and pad to meetings instead of your phone—and at night, put your phone to bed in another room so you can't check it until the morning.

WAITING FOR A DING KEEPS YOU KEYED UP.

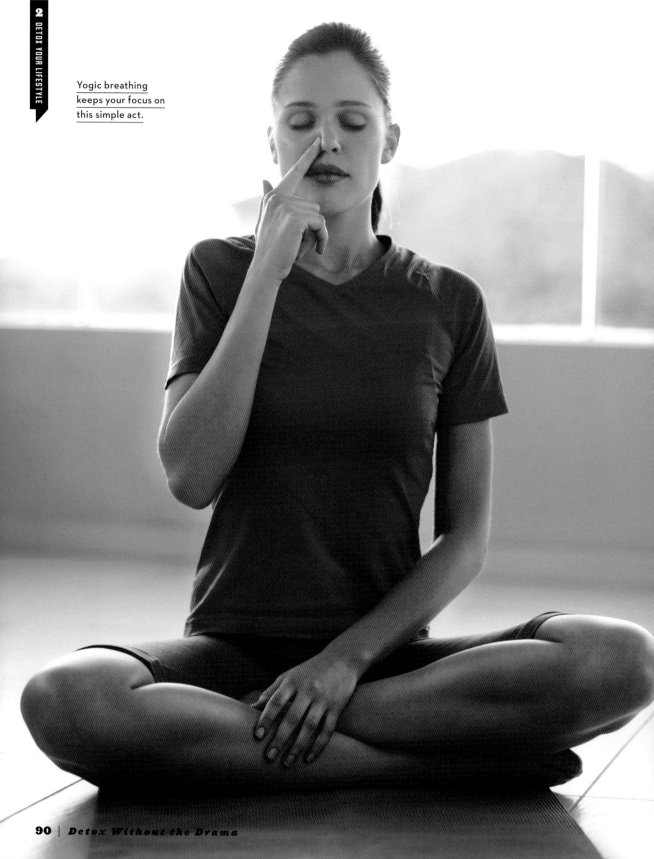

Yogic breathing
keeps your focus on
this simple act.

Mantras can help you *keep your* focus.

Headspace app, which offers what its founder calls "bite-size minis" (10-minute guided meditations); the Mindful Minute podcast, designed specifically for beginners; and the aptly named I Should Be Meditating podcast, which helps people get over any skepticism or reluctance and "just do it."

Mantra Meditation
This classic form of meditation dates back to ancient Hindu and Buddhist traditions (the earliest mantra is estimated to have been composed in Vedic Sanskrit in India more than 3,000 years ago). The use of mantras had a resurgence in the 1970s as the basis for Transcendental Meditation. It involves focusing on a word or phrase to help quiet the mind. The most basic mantra is "Om," which in Hinduism is widely known as the "Pranava mantra," the source of all mantras. You are free to use any mantra, though, or even create your own. Think of a positive affirmation that helps invite awareness into the body

and focuses you in the present moment, for example "inhale light, exhale dark" or simply "let go" (with "let" on the inhale and "go" on the exhale).

Mindfulness/Breathing Meditation
This practice allows thoughts and feelings to surface and pass without judgment or attachment, which increases awareness and acceptance of the present moment. It usually starts with a focus on the breath, counting inhalations and exhalations with a slight pause between breaths. For example, begin to slowly inhale to the count of four breaths, slightly pausing at the end of the last inhale, then lengthening the exhalation for a count of five breaths, briefly pausing at the end of the last exhale. When you feel your mind straying (and it will!), simply acknowledge the wandering and then gently bring your attention back to the breath.

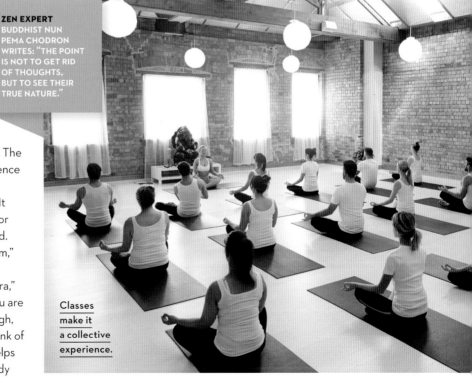

ZEN EXPERT BUDDHIST NUN PEMA CHODRON WRITES: "THE POINT IS NOT TO GET RID OF THOUGHTS, BUT TO SEE THEIR TRUE NATURE."

Classes make it a collective experience.

Detox
St★rs

THE NATURAL WORLD IS PACKED WITH POWERFUL CLEANSING AGENTS, AKA SUPERFOODS. PUT THESE ON YOUR PLATE TO CLEAR OUT TOXINS AND REBOOT YOUR MICROBIOME.

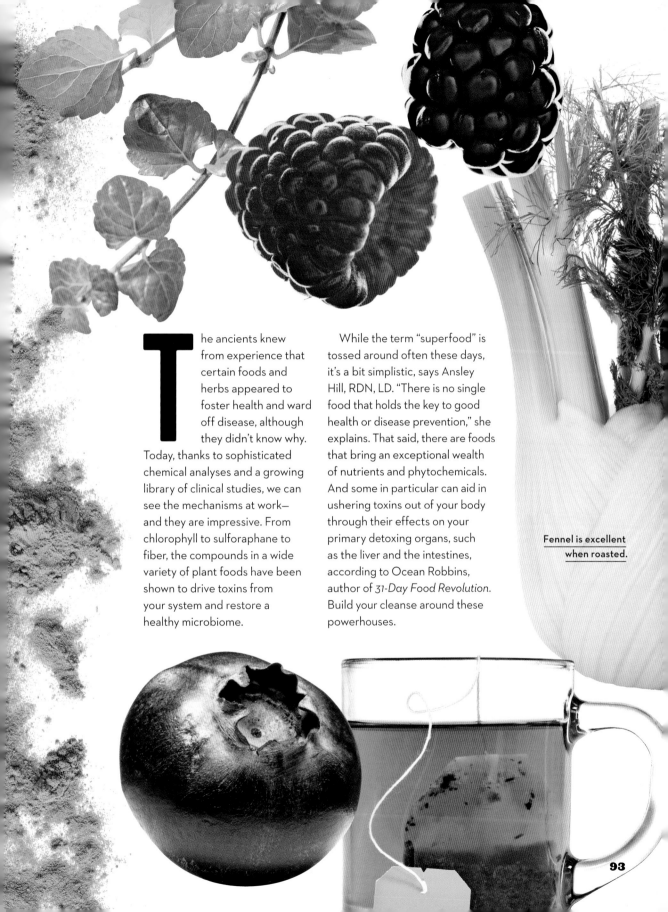

T he ancients knew from experience that certain foods and herbs appeared to foster health and ward off disease, although they didn't know why. Today, thanks to sophisticated chemical analyses and a growing library of clinical studies, we can see the mechanisms at work—and they are impressive. From chlorophyll to sulforaphane to fiber, the compounds in a wide variety of plant foods have been shown to drive toxins from your system and restore a healthy microbiome.

While the term "superfood" is tossed around often these days, it's a bit simplistic, says Ansley Hill, RDN, LD. "There is no single food that holds the key to good health or disease prevention," she explains. That said, there are foods that bring an exceptional wealth of nutrients and phytochemicals. And some in particular can aid in ushering toxins out of your body through their effects on your primary detoxing organs, such as the liver and the intestines, according to Ocean Robbins, author of *31-Day Food Revolution*. Build your cleanse around these powerhouses.

Fennel is excellent when roasted.

93

Dark, Leafy Greens

"Greens such as kale, Swiss chard, spinach and collards are excellent sources of nutrients, including folate, zinc, calcium, iron, magnesium, vitamin C and fiber," says Hill. Fiber is especially key to cleansing, both directly and indirectly. Studies show that fiber binds bile—a fluid released by the liver and stored in the gallbladder—which aids digestion, in part by breaking down waste products and facilitating their excretion. Indirectly, fiber feeds your "good" gut bacteria, some of which create short-chain fatty acids that help the liver and kidneys increase their ability to excrete toxins. Many leafy greens are also high in chlorophyll, says Robbins, which he calls "the top detoxifying plant pigment."

Root Vegetables

Many of these products of the earth—including sweet potatoes, beets, rutabagas, turnips, fennel and carrots— are packed with fiber, antioxidants and other cleansing compounds. For instance, a study in the journal *Nutrients* found that beet juice can amplify specific enzymes that support the liver and aid in detoxification. In addition, sweet potatoes have four times the RDA of the antioxidant beta-carotene, which the body converts to vitamin A, an immune-system booster (rutabagas are also rich in carotenoids). Another cleansing benefit of potatoes in general: Spuds that have been cooked and cooled are also high in resistant starch, a type of starch that passes undigested through your digestive tract and helps to feed your beneficial gut bacteria.

Cruciferous Vegetables

The cruciferous family—which includes broccoli, cauliflower, cabbage and Brussels sprouts—is high in a compound called sulforaphane. Studies show that sulforaphane can "upregulate" your liver's detoxification process and antioxidant activity, which may be one reason it also appears to lower chronic inflammation in the body. "Raw vegetables have the highest levels of sulforaphane," says dietitian Daisy Coyle, APD. "To get the most benefit, eat cruciferous vegetables raw or lightly steamed, rather than boiled or microwaved." To further boost your uptake, Coyle adds, sprinkle on some mustard seeds or mustard powder: Studies in the journals *Molecular Nutrition & Food Research* and *Food Chemistry* show that mustard can increase the bioavailability of sulforaphane, particularly in cooked vegetables, by as much as fourfold.

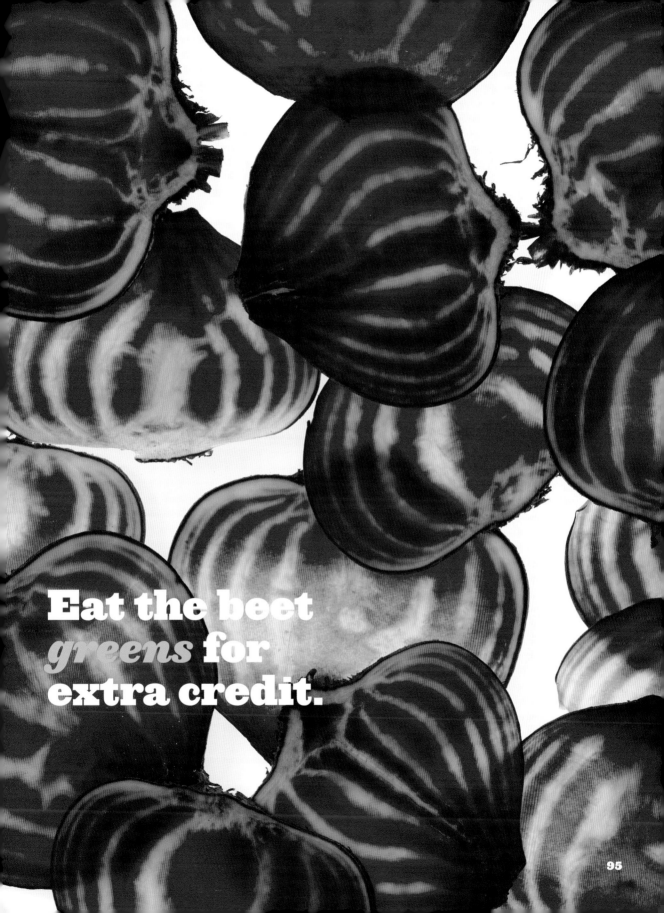

Eat the beet *greens* for extra credit.

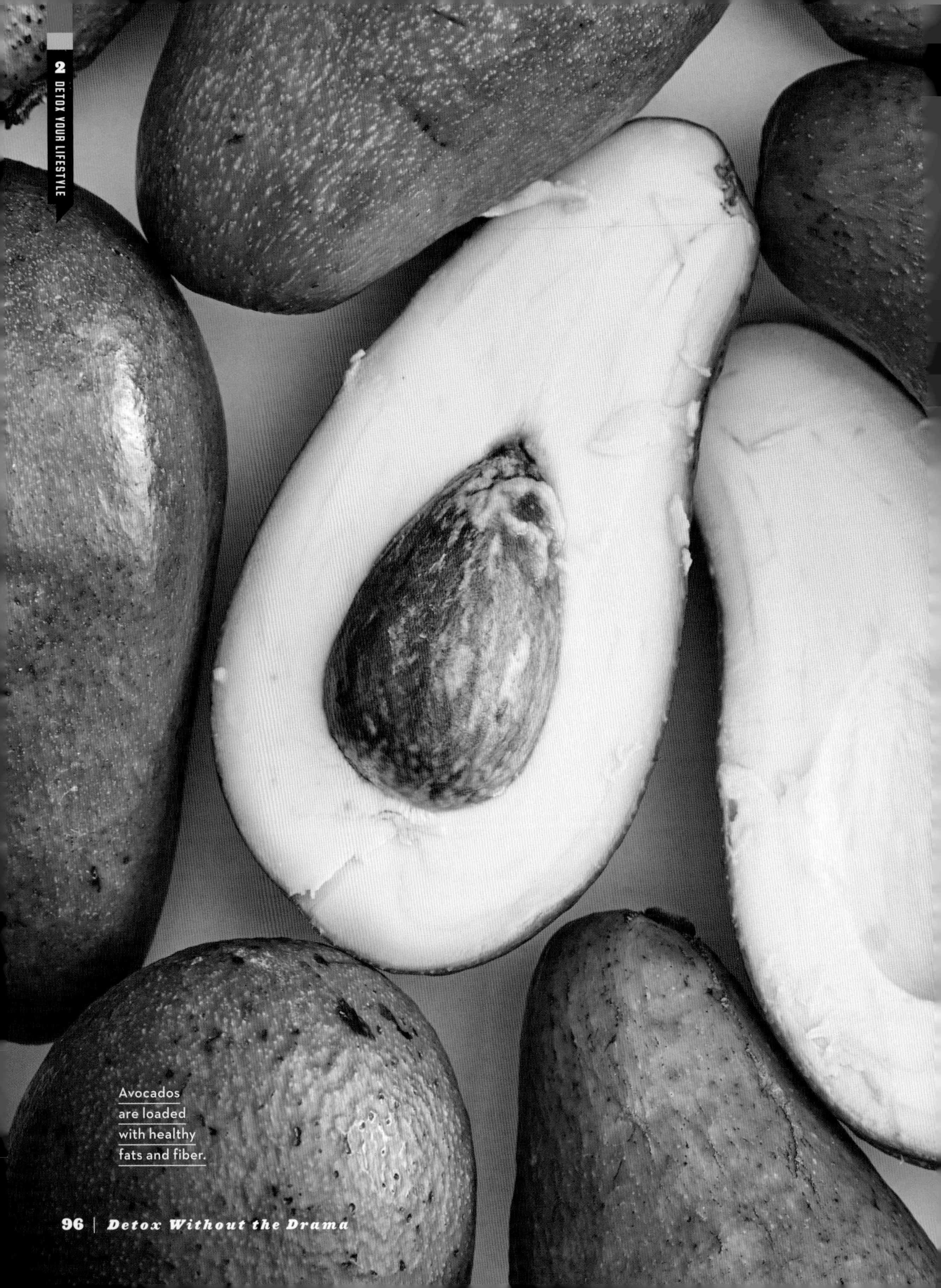

Avocados
are loaded
with healthy
fats and fiber.

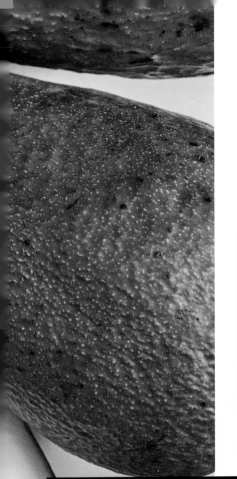

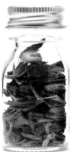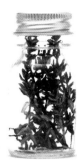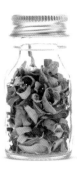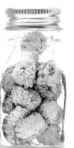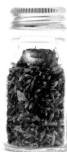

Herbs and Spices

To this day, Chinese medicine prioritizes herbs as powerful curative agents, and with good reason. Many herbs, as well as ground spices, have special detoxing properties. Take cilantro: One study found the herb can enhance mercury excretion and decrease lead absorption. "Plants that can bind to heavy metals and help your body excrete them are called 'chelators,' and cilantro is one of them," says Robbins. He also recommends turmeric, a yellow spice common in Indian cuisine that has been used medicinally for nearly 4,000 years: "[Researchers] reviewed the evidence on turmeric and found it has antibacterial, antiviral, anti-inflammatory, anti-tumor, antiseptic, cardioprotective, hepatoprotective, nephroprotective, radioprotective and digestive activities." Whew! Other cleansing herbs and spices include basil (supports the liver by increasing detoxifying enzymes and antioxidant defenses), parsley (a natural diuretic) and ginger root (its main bioactive compound is anti-inflammatory, antioxidant and aids in digestion).

In a Class of Their Own

Pop these superstars into salads, on top of yogurt or into one of the many glasses of water you should be drinking each day.

AVOCADO
This fruit is packed with healthy monounsaturated fats (similar to olive oil)—especially oleic acid, which is linked to reduced inflammation in the body—as well as fiber, vitamins and minerals. In addition, a study in the *Journal of Agricultural and Food Chemistry* found that the fatty acids in avocados help protect against damage caused by d-galactosamine, a powerful liver toxin. Mash it into guacamole or hummus, add it to salads, make it into a soup, or use it, mashed, in place of mayonnaise.

ASPARAGUS
Super high in folate and anti-inflammatories, this tasty veggie is a star in soups or salads, or as a side for supper.

BERRIES
Raspberries, strawberries, blueberries, blackberries and cranberries are all rich in nutrients and antioxidants, and promote better digestion. Put them in smoothies, salads or yogurt—or just eat them as a snack.

LEMONS
The citric acid in lemons can protect liver function and prevent oxidative damage, notes a study in the *Journal of Medicinal Food*. Another study, in the *Journal of Nutrition and Metabolism*, found that including lemon in a daily diet helped regulate blood pressure. Squeeze fresh lemon juice into water or tea, and onto salads or veggies.

Fermented Foods

These are like a gift to your gut microbiome: Fermented foods such as sauerkraut, kimchi and kombucha are loaded with good bacteria, which, in addition to their immunity-boosting powers, also help usher out heavy metals from your system. Similarly, kefir and yogurt are rich in probiotics, which feed your microbiome, the center (and in some ways the "brain") of your entire immune system.

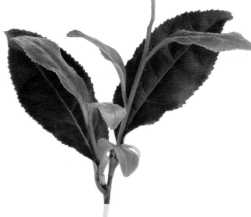

Tea

All varieties of tea are high in antioxidants, but green tea is particularly rich in compounds that are also anti-inflammatory. "One of the most prevalent antioxidants in green tea is epigallocatechin gallate (EGCG)," says Hill. "This compound is likely what gives green tea its apparent ability to protect against chronic diseases, including heart disease, diabetes and cancer." Research also shows that the combination of catechins and caffeine in green tea can help some people burn fat and lose weight. Matcha, a green tea powder, is especially high in EGCG, as well as chlorophyll. A study in the journal *Cancer Epidemiology, Biomarkers & Prevention* found that matcha boosted production of detoxification enzymes, which play a key role in cancer prevention. Drink it hot or iced.

How Important Is Organic?

It can't hurt! But don't panic if you can't always eat (or afford) organic, say experts.

It's clear that eating a whole-food, largely plant-based diet is an important part of detoxing your entire system and promoting optimal health. But that raises the inevitable question: What about pesticides and other toxins that may be used in raising those plants (as well as in raising livestock)? In a perfect world, we would all eat farm-raised, pesticide-free foods all the time, but that's not always feasible.

"It's ideal to choose sustainably raised—grass-fed, and hormone- and antibiotic-free—animal products and to choose organic fruits and vegetables," says Melissa Young, MD, an integrative and functional medicine specialist at the Cleveland Clinic. "But if that's not possible, it's still highly recommended to eat nine to 11 servings of fruits and vegetables daily—of diverse color and variety—to obtain your phytonutrients and antioxidants." Her suggestions: Wash produce well, peel fruits and vegetables that don't have a thick skin, and prioritize your organic spending for items that are listed on the Environmental Working Group's "Dirty Dozen" list. That's the EWG's annual list of fruits and vegetables that test highest for pesticides (ewg.org). The good news: The USDA has found that the vast majority of foods contain either no detectable residues, or residues that are below limits set by the Environmental Protection Agency.

Nuts and Seeds

These little treats are bundles of fiber, healthy fats (including omega-3s, in some cases) and anti-inflammatory compounds. Seeds such as hemp, flax and chia are not only rich in antioxidants, but their high fiber content helps cleanse the colon and facilitate toxin removal. Numerous studies have shown a heart-protective effect of both nuts and seeds, says Hill, and even though they tend to be calorie-dense, "some types of nuts are linked to weight loss when included in a balanced diet." Look for almonds, pecans, pistachios, walnuts, cashews, Brazil nuts and macadamias, as well as a variety of seeds (including all of those listed above).

Big things come in small packages—such as nuts and seeds.

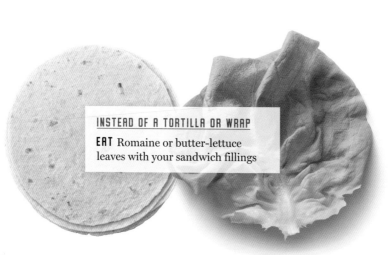

INSTEAD OF A TORTILLA OR WRAP

EAT Romaine or butter-lettuce leaves with your sandwich fillings

Smart Food Swaps

Eating clean doesn't have to mean missing your favorite flavors and textures. Try these easy, tasty hacks.

Everyone has a jones for ice cream, chips or other commercially made treats once in a while. Luckily, it turns out you don't have to cave—you can whip up something at home that rivals your old, unhealthy go-tos.

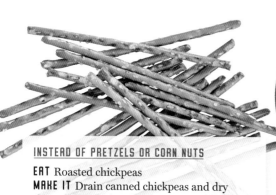

INSTEAD OF PRETZELS OR CORN NUTS

EAT Roasted chickpeas
MAKE IT Drain canned chickpeas and dry them well, drizzle with olive oil and salt, and cook in a 400 F oven for 20 to 30 minutes until browned, shaking the pan every 10 minutes. Sprinkle with your favorite spices (try garlic powder, curry or chili powder).

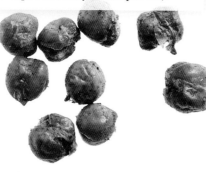

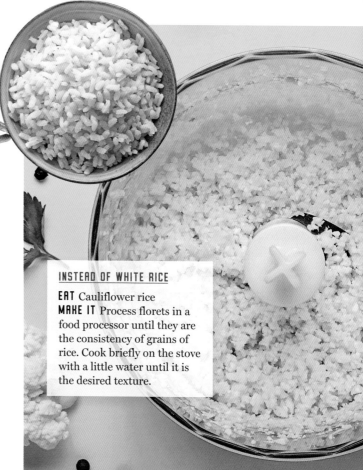

INSTEAD OF WHITE RICE

EAT Cauliflower rice
MAKE IT Process florets in a food processor until they are the consistency of grains of rice. Cook briefly on the stove with a little water until it is the desired texture.

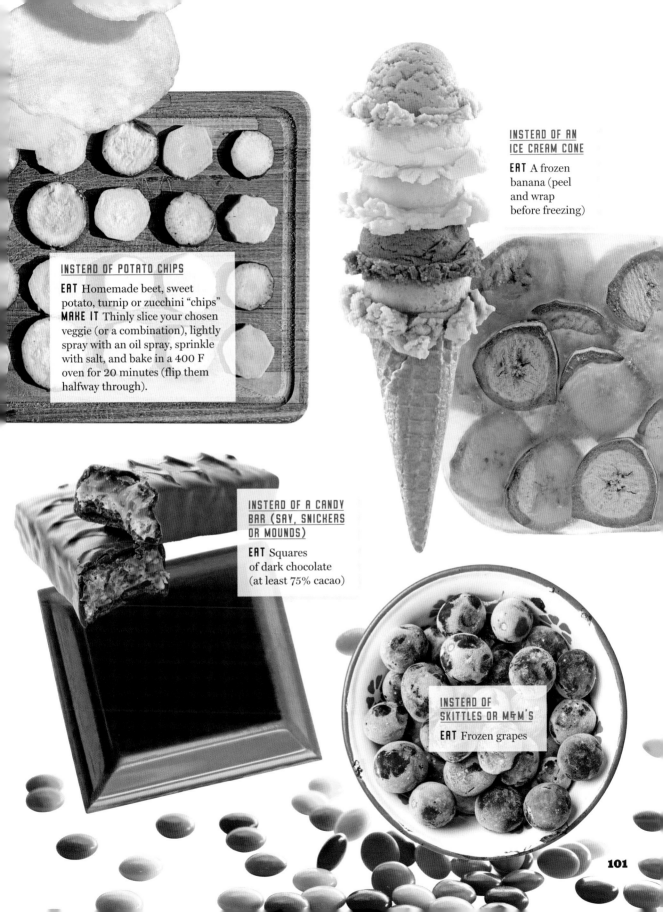

INSTEAD OF POTATO CHIPS

EAT Homemade beet, sweet potato, turnip or zucchini "chips"
MAKE IT Thinly slice your chosen veggie (or a combination), lightly spray with an oil spray, sprinkle with salt, and bake in a 400 F oven for 20 minutes (flip them halfway through).

INSTEAD OF AN ICE CREAM CONE

EAT A frozen banana (peel and wrap before freezing)

INSTEAD OF A CANDY BAR (SAY, SNICKERS OR MOUNDS)

EAT Squares of dark chocolate (at least 75% cacao)

INSTEAD OF SKITTLES OR M&M'S

EAT Frozen grapes

101

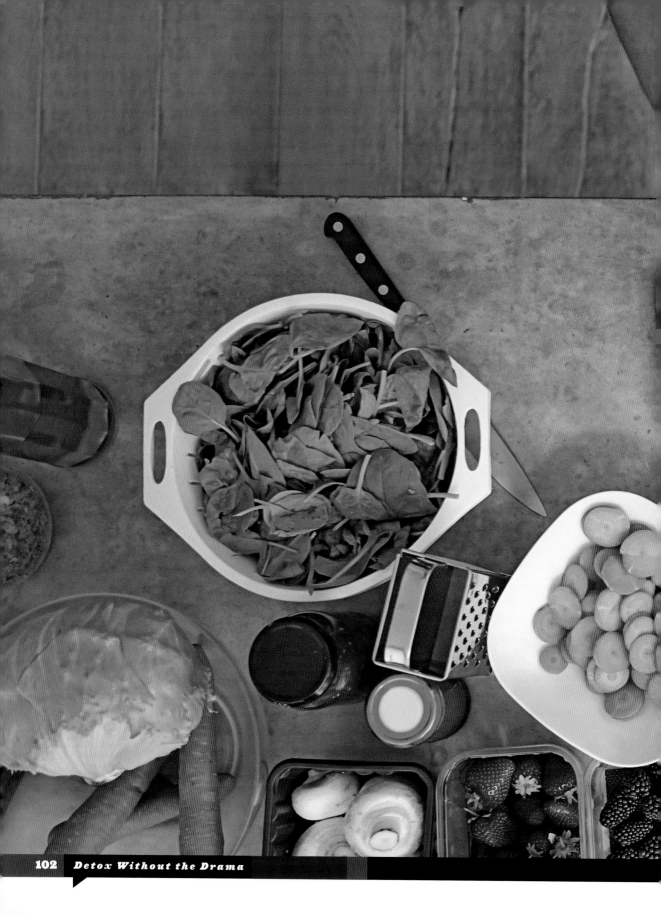

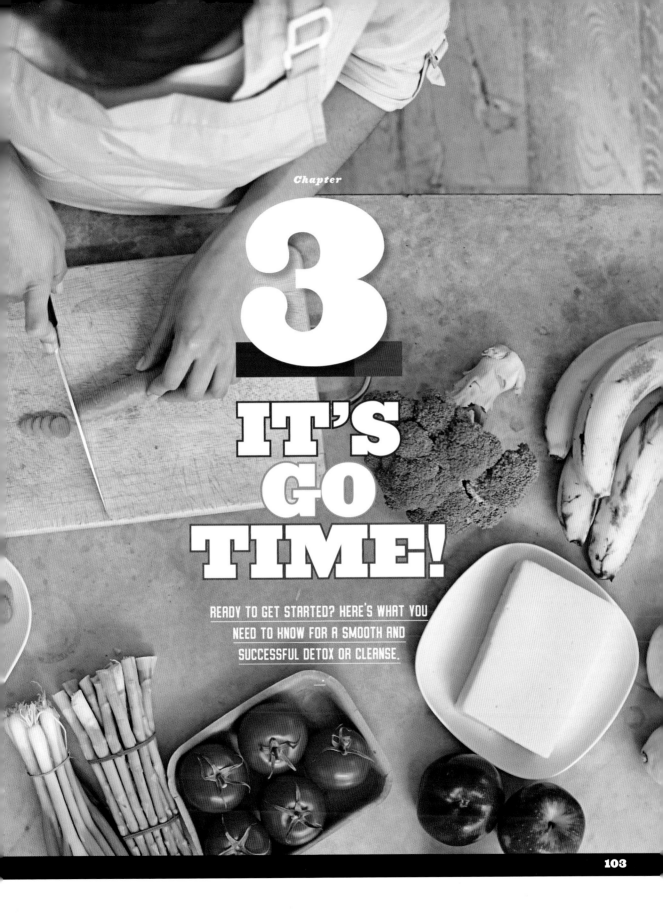

3

IT'S GO TIME!

READY TO GET STARTED? HERE'S WHAT YOU
NEED TO KNOW FOR A SMOOTH AND
SUCCESSFUL DETOX OR CLEANSE.

Get a Head Start

GEARING UP FOR YOUR CLEANSE,
BUT NOT QUITE READY? HERE ARE 10 THINGS YOU CAN
DO TODAY TO GET THE BALL ROLLING.

You've been doing your research and figuring out which program will work best for you, because you want to do your cleanse right. But if you're impatient, you can begin making these changes right now.

1 Take a Sauna

"A study analyzed the sweat of people whose bodies had tested higher for toxins and heavy metals, and it was loaded with toxins that had been excreted," says Peter Bennett, ND, co-author of *7-Day Detox Miracle*. When you get your sweat on at your leisure in a dry or steam sauna, you begin to understand the thinking behind sweat lodges and other ancient practices—and emerge with smooth skin and refreshed circulation.

2 Hit the Shower

Bennett prescribes this as the hydrotherapy part of his seven-day detox program, and says it helps the flow of blood and lymph through the organs, especially the intestines. "As blood travels in and out of these areas, it delivers nutrients and takes away cellular waste products, and also enhances the activity of the immune system." His method: Take a hot shower for five minutes, switch to cold for 30 seconds, then repeat the cycle two more times. Dry off, get in bed for 30 minutes and stay warm.

3 Make a Detox Viewing List

There are a slew of films documenting aspects of our food industry and environment that will give you motivation for starting your cleanse. Check out: *Fat, Sick & Nearly Dead; Forks Over Knives; Hungry For Change; Food, Inc.; Food Matters; Super Size Me;* and *Cooked.*

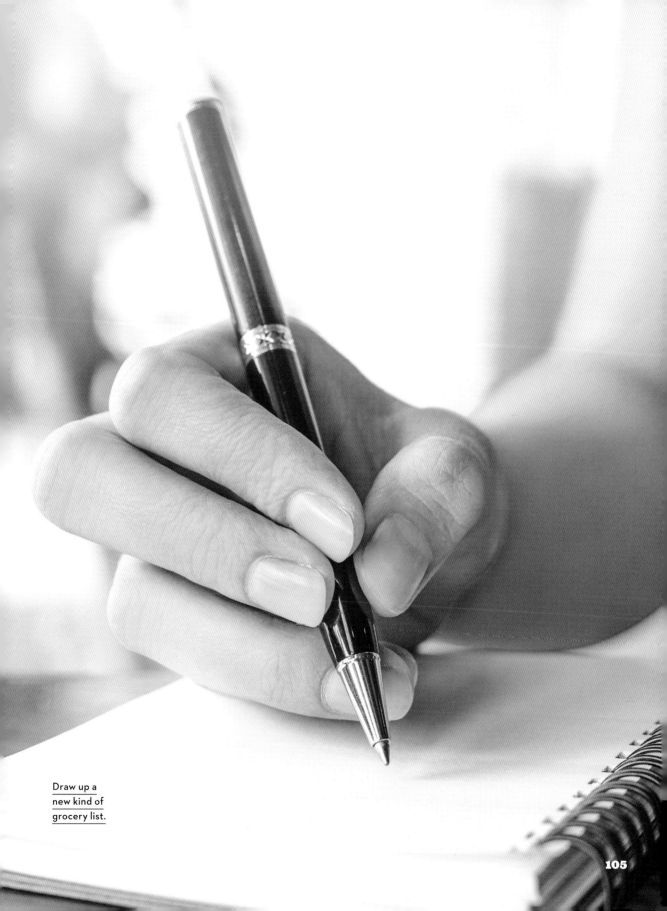

Draw up a
new kind of
grocery list.

Beans are nutrition powerhouses.

4 Eat Beans

They're packed with soluble fiber, which starts the detox process in two ways: Directly, it binds bile and the toxins it collects and ushers them out of the body; indirectly, it feeds the bacteria in your digestive tract, some of which create short-chain fatty acids and other metabolites that help the liver and kidneys excrete toxins. Other top fiber sources include bran, barley, citrus fruits, peas, legumes and potatoes.

5 Take a Before Picture

And measure your body. If your cleanse ends up being a game-changer, you'll be sorry you didn't!

6 Dry-Brush Your Skin

Another ancient ritual that has made a comeback, dry-brushing improves your skin's role in detoxification by exfoliating, removing dead skin and possibly helping the lymph system move toxins out of your system. Use a natural-bristle brush made for the purpose (you can find them on Amazon) and gently but firmly brush your skin in long strokes toward your heart. Then shower and apply a vitamin-rich moisturizer to your skin.

7 Download a Meditation App

Starting a practice is challenging—but it's key to the body-mind impact of your cleanse. Get some guidance from apps that talk you through the process, including: The Mindfulness App, which offers guides from three to 30 minutes long; Calm, with exercises and breathing techniques to help you relax; and Aura, which starts with three-minute sessions.

8 Ease Off Caffeine

Most cleanses suggest ditching caffeine, so if you're a java junkie, lower your intake now to avoid suffering through withdrawal headaches later. Green tea (with a small amount of caffeine) is usually OK in detox, or go right to water with lemon juice.

9 Find a Detox Buddy

Cleansing with a friend can set you up for success in all kinds of ways. You can share tips and help each other stick to the plan in moments of temptation, and it helps to know you're not alone in your plan.

10 Shop Organic

Studies show that switching from conventional to organic produce can reduce biomarkers of organophosphate-class pesticides in as little as a week. There's also evidence that organic foods have more beneficial nutrients, including antioxidants, than conventionally grown fare. Tops on the list of most pesticide-laden fare are strawberries, spinach, kale, nectarines, apples, grapes, cherries, peaches, pears and bell or hot peppers.

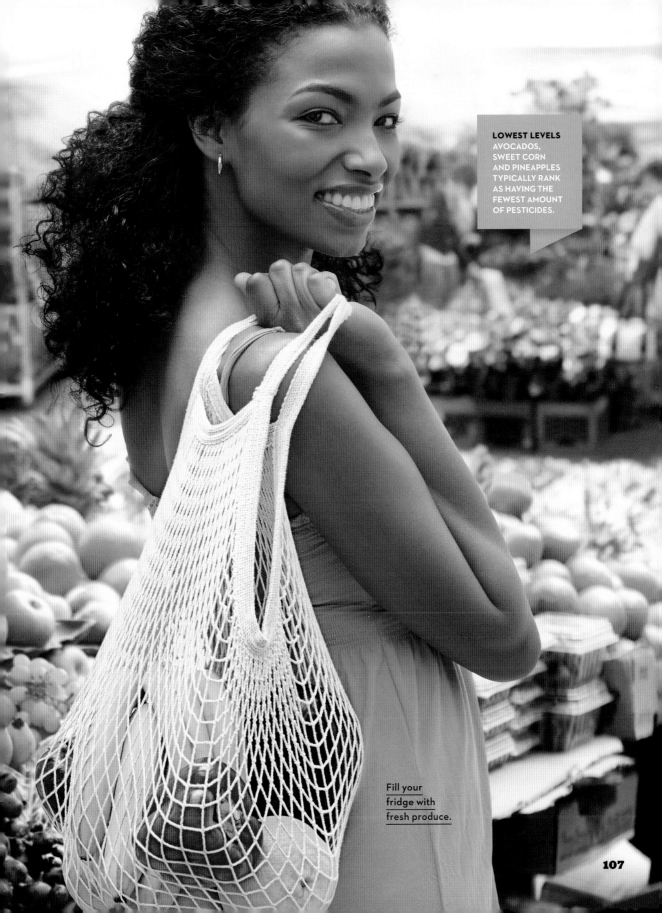

LOWEST LEVELS
AVOCADOS, SWEET CORN AND PINEAPPLES TYPICALLY RANK AS HAVING THE FEWEST AMOUNT OF PESTICIDES.

Fill your fridge with fresh produce.

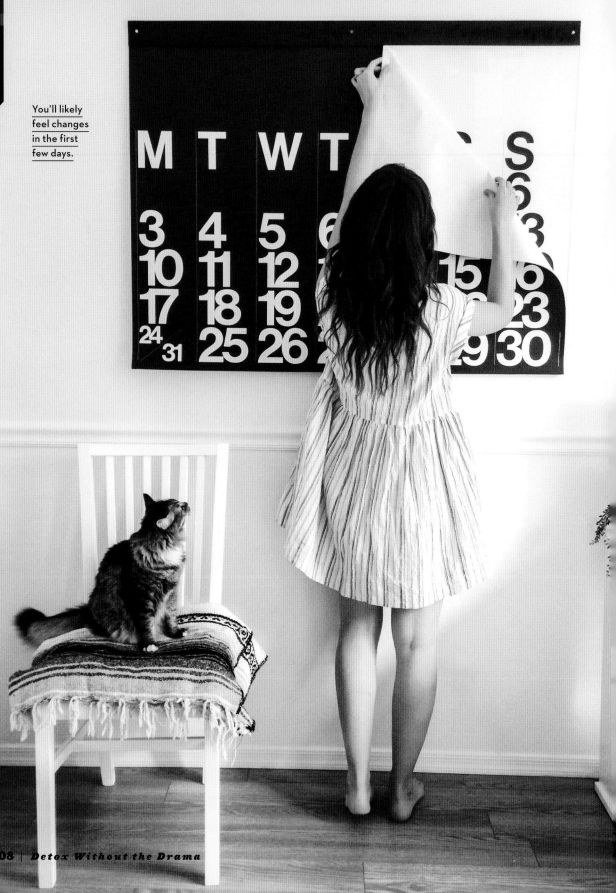

You'll likely feel changes in the first few days.

Kick Off Your Cleanse

LAUNCHING WHAT YOU HOPE WILL BE A LIFE-CHANGING DETOX? HERE'S HOW TO MAKE THE MOST OF IT FROM THE START.

When you hear the word "cleanse," do you imagine existing on liquids only for days, or choking down pricey supplements? That's an outdated notion of cleansing that typically leads only to short-term gains. Instead, picture this: Give yourself two weeks of eliminating all common allergens—dairy, eggs, gluten, sugar, corn, nightshades, soy, caffeine and alcohol—and replace them with nutrient-dense whole foods such as non-gluten grains, nuts, seeds, dark, leafy greens and organic lean meats (if you eat meat) or plant proteins. No counting calories—just eating when you're hungry and tuning in to how you feel.

Jo Schaalman and Julie Peláez, creators of the popular Conscious Cleanse program, say it only takes one to two weeks to see a change. After that, you'll have less chronic inflammation—and a clean slate. You can choose to reintroduce foods to your diet systematically, and figure out the foods your body likes best. Research has shown that there's no "one-size-fits-all" approach to eating—some people thrive as omnivores, others feel tip-top on a vegan diet, and many of us have hidden food sensitivities that a two-week cleanse will help to identify. Read on for a primer on prepping for a cleanse and how to make the most of your first few days on a plan.

Clean Eating Essentials

The word "cleanse" comes, of course, from the word "clean." That means mostly choosing whole foods in their natural form, and avoiding highly processed, packaged foods. Focus on foods that are minimally processed, free of chemicals and close to the way they appear in nature. If there's an ingredient you can't pronounce, don't eat it. To start cleansing, first stock up on these five must-haves for your fridge:

Lots of Veggies

Vegetables are the center of a clean-eater's universe. Opt for leafy greens (kale, spinach, chard, collards, etc.) you can use multiple ways—such as in meals and smoothies. Grab other veggies you can slice and eat as snacks or toss in salads. Good choices include cucumbers, radishes, carrots, celery and avocados.

Nut Milk

Have a high-quality nut milk on hand at all times; nut milk is a key ingredient for many of the recipes starting in Chapter 4 (see page 150), especially the smoothies. The best choice is to make your own. If that's not an option, store-bought milk will work, but be a label detective. Many nut milks include ingredients such as carrageenan, guar gum, natural flavors, citric acid, or vegetable oils that you should avoid. Look for best brands such as like Malk and Forager Project. If you are allergic to nuts, try hempseed, avocado, rice or coconut milk.

Dressing or Dip
Having a tasty salad dressing or dip on hand throughout the week can make a big difference in your meal prep. The cleanest option is to make your own, with simple ingredients such as pureed vegetables and/or oil and vinegar. If you do need to buy a dip or dressing, look for as few ingredients as possible, and avoid additives and preservatives such as guar gum, xanthan gum and citric acid, and allergens such as peanuts, soybean oil, gluten or dairy.

Animal or Plant Protein
Have a prepared animal or plant protein on hand to use in a salad or bowl. If you're going for plant protein, look for chickpeas, lentils, beans, nuts such as walnuts or almonds, or seeds such as pumpkin or hempseeds. Try to buy organic, and if you're buying canned beans make sure they have no added ingredients and are BPA-free. For animal protein, look for lean, organic, free-range meat—such as chicken, lamb, bison or turkey—and/or wild-caught fish, such as cod, salmon or trout.

Whole Grains
Having a cooked batch of rice, quinoa, millet or buckwheat on hand can make meal prep a breeze. When shopping, look for organic, non-gluten grains. Avoid precooked rice packets or boxed grain blends that have high sodium levels or artificial additives (read labels to check).

Plan Your Meal
The baseline of cleanses such as the Conscious Cleanse eating plan consists of filling two-thirds of your plate with veggies, supplemented with a protein or a non-gluten grain. **Here's how to construct a typical meal:**

4 to 8 ounces animal or vegetable protein OR 1 to 2 cups non-gluten grain (for the healthiest food combo, choose protein or grain, not both)

Unlimited raw or lightly steamed vegetables, plus fruits; 1 or 2 tablespoons healthy oil (olive, borage, flaxseed, hempseed; sesame and coconut when cooking)

Drink lots of water.

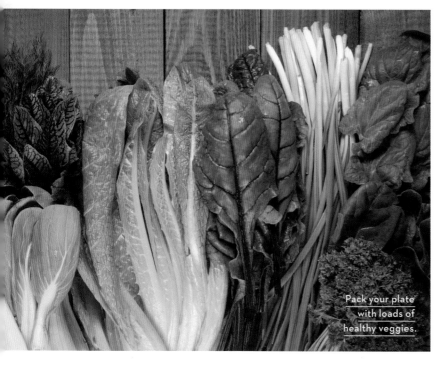

Pack your plate with loads of healthy veggies.

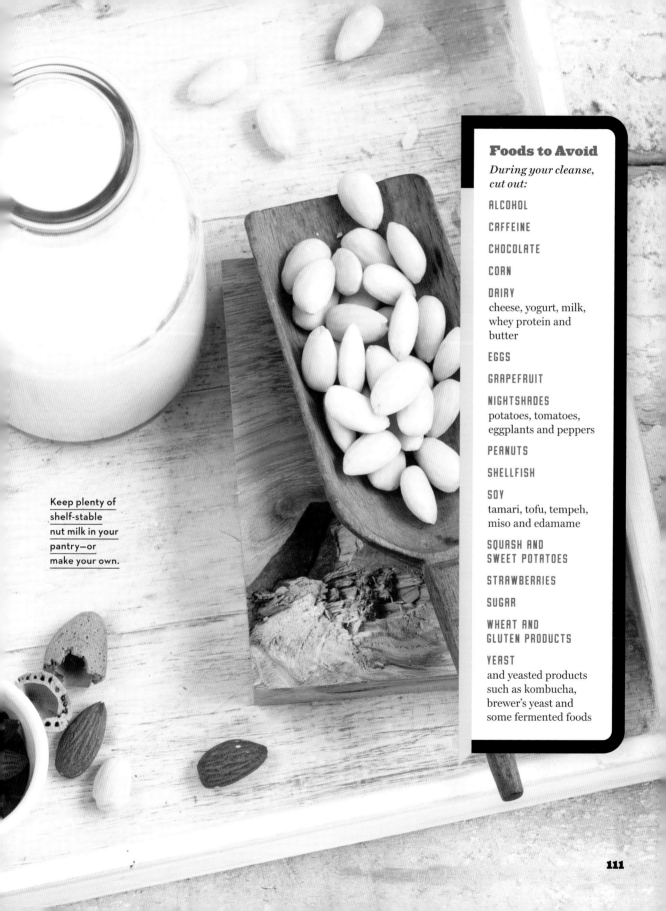

Keep plenty of shelf-stable nut milk in your pantry—or make your own.

Foods to Avoid

During your cleanse, cut out:

ALCOHOL

CAFFEINE

CHOCOLATE

CORN

DAIRY
cheese, yogurt, milk, whey protein and butter

EGGS

GRAPEFRUIT

NIGHTSHADES
potatoes, tomatoes, eggplants and peppers

PEANUTS

SHELLFISH

SOY
tamari, tofu, tempeh, miso and edamame

SQUASH AND SWEET POTATOES

STRAWBERRIES

SUGAR

WHEAT AND GLUTEN PRODUCTS

YEAST
and yeasted products such as kombucha, brewer's yeast and some fermented foods

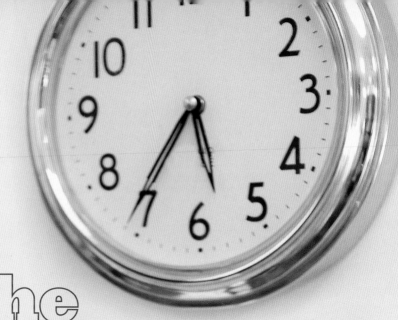

The Fast

GOING WITHOUT FOOD
FOR CERTAIN PERIODS OF TIME,
FROM HOURS TO A DAY
OR MORE, IS ONE OF THE MOST
EFFICIENT WAYS TO GIVE
YOUR WHOLE BODY A
HEALTH-BOOSTING CLEANSE.

All you have
to do is watch
the clock.

What if you could help your body repair and refresh—and even lose some weight—just by rearranging your eating schedule?

That's what more and more evidence is showing that intermittent fasting (IF) can do:

to detoxing. "As humans, we're fully wired for fasting," says Peter Bennett, ND, co-author of *7-Day Detox Miracle*. "Our physiology is all set up to go for periods of time without eating." In fact, Bennett says, "our bodies kind of like it." Describing the traditional Buddhist monks' vow to eat once a day at noon, he adds: "People have been doing

Why Fasting Is Cleansing

Many cultures and religions have traditionally practiced some form of fasting: Muslims during Ramadan, Jews during Yom Kippur, Christians during Lent, and the Buddhist monks that Bennett mentions, who fast for much of each day. The ancients appeared to recognize

Solution

reduce inflammation, clear out cellular detritus, promote healthy replacement-cell growth, improve your metabolic processes— and overall, give your natural detoxification systems a break from digestive duties so they can concentrate on clearing out other accumulated toxins. A study in the prestigious *New England Journal of Medicine* concluded that "intermittent fasting elicits evolutionarily conserved, adaptive cellular responses that... suppress inflammation."

Intermittent fasting, which can take many forms, has been gaining traction as both a weight-loss aid and a health-promoting intervention for several years now. And certain aspects of IF have become increasingly viewed as central

intermittent fasting in ancient cultures for thousands of years." What modern science shows, says Bennett, is that IF can be a reboot of your whole system, "like pressing the reset button on your computer."

Why would simply skipping breakfast and eating between noon and 8 p.m., or taking a single day (or two) off from eating, have such a profound effect on your inherent detoxification systems? The answer lies, in part, with your body's innate natural detox abilities, how they interact with the food you eat—and how humans have eaten for most of our history. Read on for a short course in how to fast safely.

that fasting had special benefits, including mental clarity. Plato proclaimed, "I fast for greater physical and mental efficiency," and Buddha is believed to have reached his enlightenment through fasting. Now, using advanced scientific tools, we have begun to understand why. One reason is a phenomenon called autophagy (Greek for "self-eating"), which is your body's inherent way of cleansing the cells and clearing out damaged bits and pieces. Over time, through the processes of daily living, your cells accumulate a variety of oxidized particles, dead organelles and damaged proteins, which can "gunk

CLEARHEADED INTERMITTENT FASTING IS SHOWN TO IMPROVE MENTAL CLARITY BY HELPING CLEAR CELLULAR DEBRIS FROM THE BRAIN.

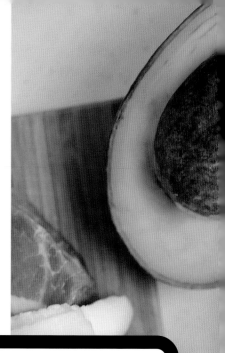

up" your system. The result: inflammation and an acceleration of the aging process, because those clogging particles can prevent the cells from dividing and functioning normally. Autophagy is like the nighttime garbageman who sweeps through your body and clears out the cellular trash.

The problem is that when you eat, the increased levels of proteins, glucose and insulin (which is released to break down the glucose) all switch off autophagy. "By eating constantly, from the time we wake up to the time we sleep, we prevent the activation of autophagy's cleansing pathways," says Jason Fung, MD, the author of *The Complete Guide to Fasting*. "Simply put, fasting cleanses the body of unhealthy or unnecessary cellular debris."

The Total Body Benefits of Fasting

Your organs, bloodstream, hormones, even your mitochondria—the energy factories within each cell—respond to every period of fasting you go through. IF allows key parts of your immune system, digestive system and natural detoxing process to rest from processing food and just cleanse your body. Here's how that works, from head to toe.

BRAIN
Studies show that IF can prompt growth of new neurons and signaling pathways, a process called neuroplasticity, especially in the hippocampus (the center of learning and memory). The autophagy that comes with IF also clears out dying or damaged cells and toxic proteins from the brain, helping to deter dementia.

HEART
Inflammation is strongly linked to cardiovascular disease, so the anti-inflammatory effects of IF help keep arteries clear of buildup.

LYMPHATIC SYSTEM
This organ system is part of both the circulatory and immune systems, and works as a filter for the blood, carrying out waste and cellular debris while mounting an immune defense. Giving it a rest from cleansing related to food gives it more freedom to move out toxins.

LIVER
Virtually everything that goes through your body—food, alcohol, medicine, toxins—is routed through the liver, the heart of your detoxing system. When freed from its work on food and drink, the liver steps up its cleansing job on various toxins, whether from the environment or from the natural by-products of cell function, and flushes them out.

WAISTLINE
Many people start a cleanse hoping to drop pounds, and studies show that people on IF lose weight and have a lower body mass index. That's because after fasting for 12 hours, you start burning stored fat instead of food. IF is especially good at reducing abdominal fat, the most dangerous kind—it can release toxins into nearby organs.

JOINTS
Many joint issues, including rheumatoid arthritis, are tied to inflammation. The systemic drop in inflammation that results from periods of fasting can quickly reduce pain and help protect your joints.

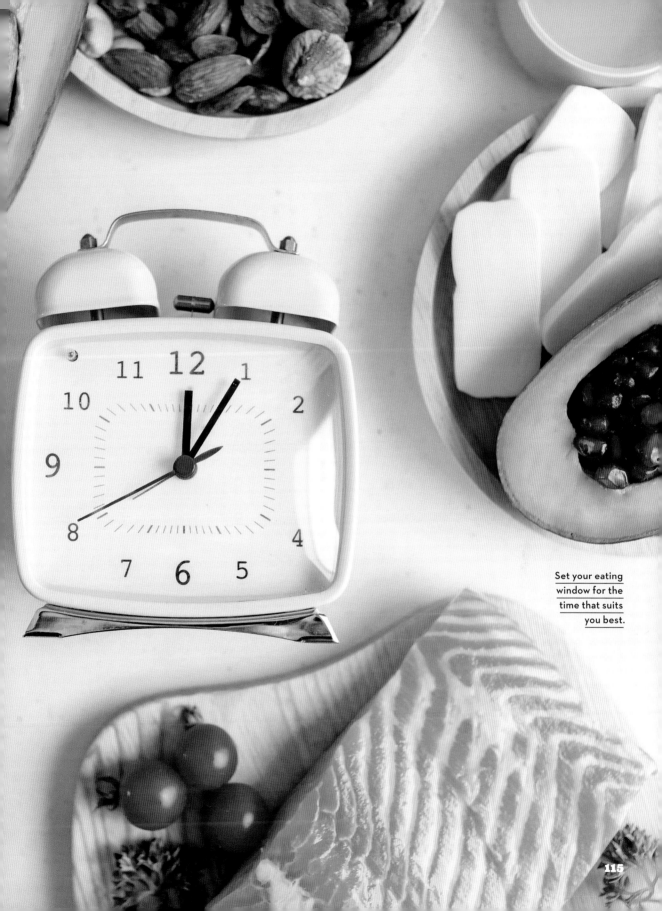

Set your eating window for the time that suits you best.

Try breaking
your fast with
a smoothie.

Fasting also affects your reticuloendothelial system (RES), which consists of cells whose main function is to remove dead or abnormal cells, tissues and foreign substances, says Bennett. The RES includes the liver and also the spleen and lymphoid organs, and is a key part of your immune system. When you stop eating, your RES is freed up to concentrate solely on clearing out toxic substances and cell particles.

"Your liver is like a massive processing center," explains Bennett. "It assembles molecules, rips them apart, stores them, assembles hormone precursors." But the liver also must process the fats, sugars and proteins you ingest. "While it's dealing with food, it's also constantly cleaning the blood of the 'metabolic sweat' of every cell in your body." Take food out of the equation, Bennett says, "and the liver gets to play catch-up on all this assembling and disassembling. The longer you rest the liver from food, the cleaner your blood's going to be. Based on this physiology, intermittent fasting is a good idea." That's why Bennett's seven-day detox program starts with a two-day water fast, and why he advises that, whatever program you follow, "Once a year, stop eating for two days." That may

ANCIENT WISDOM HOMO SAPIENS EVOLVED TO THRIVE THROUGH PERIODS OF FAMINE AND DEPRIVATION—NOT A LIFESTYLE OF CONSTANT EATING.

An IF no-no: Don't binge on fried food!

sound draconian to some people, though. Luckily, several different forms of IF have become popular in the last decade or so—and some may be easier for many people to follow.

Take Your Pick

There are essentially four ways to fast intermittently, so you can "shop" for the system that's right for you. One thing they all share (in addition to being effective for health and weight loss), is the premise that when you *do* eat, you must prioritize healthy, microbiome-boosting foods.

That doesn't mean that your eating periods are like a diet, and in fact it's counterproductive to try to undereat as well as fast—you'll just end up ditching the plan. You can eat to satiation during your eating window, but don't consider it a free pass to binge on ice cream or a host of fried foods. Concentrate on a well-rounded diet that includes plenty of leafy greens, colorful fruits and vegetables, whole grains, legumes, nuts and seeds, and organic, grass-fed or wild proteins. Consider the following styles of intermittent fasting.

16:8 or Time-Restricted Feeding

This IF pattern involves taking in all your calories within a daily window of time, usually eight hours (although some people shorten the window to six hours). Many people find this the easiest IF plan to stick to, because it's not far off from a "normal" eating schedule. The most common form is to skip breakfast, have your first meal at noon, and finish dinner by 8 p.m. It's also quite flexible, as long as you maintain your window, and some early risers prefer to follow a 10 a.m. to 6 p.m. schedule. Within your window, just eat healthy meals until you're full, without counting calories.

5:2 or Alternate-Day Fasting

This may be the most-studied form of IF, having been tested in numerous studies. In 5:2, you fast for one full day twice a week (most people choose Monday and Thursday), and in alternate-day fasting you fast every other day. The "fast days" do allow a small number of calories, usually 500 to 600, so you can eat a hard-boiled egg, for instance, and a simple salad with a small serving of tuna or chicken. While some fasters find this method too demanding, others like the simplicity of the all-or-nothing approach. After your fast day, you can enjoy a full day of regular, healthy meals.

3 Keys to Success

Experts and experienced time-restricted eaters agree that following these simple guidelines will make your 16:8 plan easier.

1 LEAN TOWARD LOW-CARB

An important part of IF is dealing with hunger—and eating a higher-fat, lower-carb diet will make hunger less of an issue. Many studies show a high-fat diet is more satiating than a low-carb one. So breaking your fast with a higher-fat (and moderate protein) meal, or ending your day with one, may make the next day easier to handle.

2 DON'T UNDEREAT

Do not try to lower or slash your calorie intake at the same time as doing IF. The whole point of IF is that you can eat "normally" (whatever that means to you) because it's about timing, not calorie-counting. Even more importantly, if you don't eat enough during your eating window, you'll be too hungry to stick to the program.

3 FORGIVE YOURSELF

This is a lifestyle, not a diet. To do 16:8 over the long term, you must accept that every now and then you'll have a day that doesn't fit the plan. It could happen during the holidays, at a stressful moment, during a busy time or while traveling and/or on vacation. Just return to the schedule when you can—and think "marathon," not "sprint."

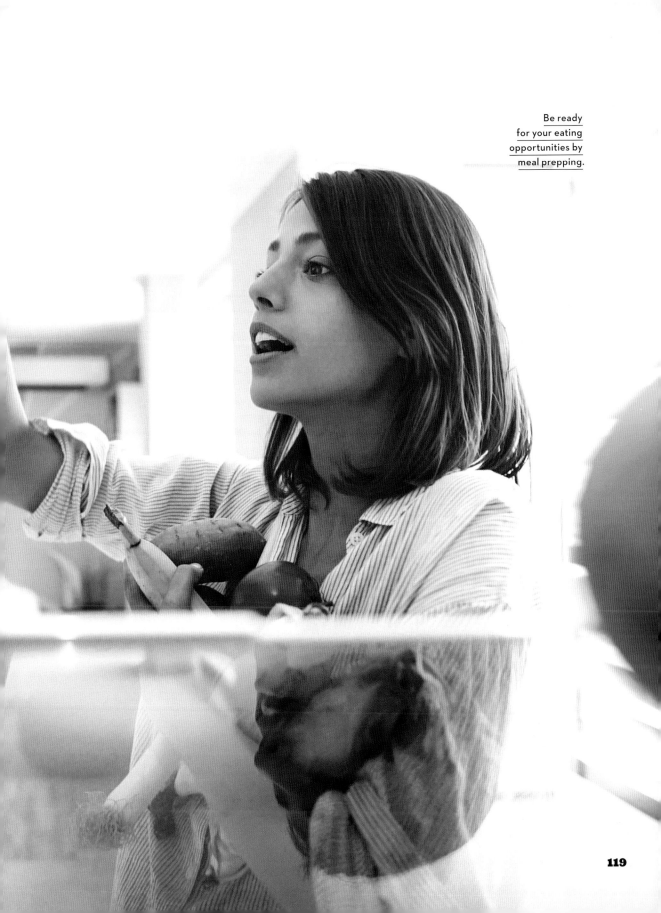

Be ready
for your eating
opportunities by
meal prepping.

Make your
first meal
after a fast a
delicious one.

Fasting makes the *food* you do eat more vital.

One Meal a Day (OMAD) or Warrior

On Warrior, you fast most of the day (although some people also munch on a few raw veggies) and then eat one big meal. This cuts your eating window down to two to three hours tops. For some that sounds counterintuitive—don't nutritionists always tell us to "eat breakfast like a king, lunch like a prince and dinner like a pauper"? But the science of IF shows that abstaining from food for more than 12 hours burns fat and speeds the metabolism. The problem with late-night eating (without being on Warrior) is more likely that people tend to nosh on junk-food snacks or desserts late in the day, and that they have been eating regular meals all day long, resulting in an overall calorie overload (and never giving their system a chance to cleanse and repair).

Extended Fasts

Anything over 24 hours is an extended fast. Within these parameters, though, there are choices. For instance, instead of going from dinner to the next day's dinner (24 hours), you could eat dinner, fast for the following day, and eat breakfast on the third day (36 hours). If you push breakfast to noon on day three, that's 42 hours. Extended fasters can drink liquids with a few calories, like bone broth. Benefits accrue quickly on this plan, says Fung, but there's a higher risk of complications, so he advises consulting your doctor first.

True or False?

Setting the record straight on misconceptions about intermittent fasting.

MYTH 1
GOING WITHOUT FOOD SLOWS YOUR METABOLISM
REALITY Fasting instead raises your basal metabolism, burning more calories, says Jason Fung, MD. It's true that traditional diets do slow metabolism —that's a big reason most dieters regain weight. In long-term restriction, your body learns how to subsist on fewer calories for survival. But when you eat zero food for a period, your metabolism can't also go to zero, so your body switches its energy source from food to stored body fat, says Fung. Studies show an increase in fat-burning during a fast.

MYTH 2
FASTING CAUSES LOW BLOOD SUGAR
REALITY Glucose from the breakdown of food is the body's most easily accessed fuel, but we can energize our bodies in other ways, too. When you run out of glucose in short-term storage (called glycogen), your liver breaks down stored fat into a usable form, called ketones. (This also happens as a result of the keto diet.) So you won't turn into a shaky, light-headed mess when fasting, says Fung; you'll just continue to function on a different energy source.

MYTH 3
FASTING IS LIKE STARVING
REALITY The difference between the two is pretty clear, says Fung: One is a choice, and one is involuntary. "It's the difference between recreational running, and running because a lion is chasing you."

MYTH 4
YOU'LL BINGE WHEN YOU BREAK YOUR FAST
REALITY Studies show that people do eat a little more after they have been fasting, but it's typically only a few hundred calories—not a binge, and still much less than you would likely have taken in if you had been eating every few hours. "And with repeated fasting, appetite tends to decrease as the fasting duration continues," says Fung. Of course, like anything, you can easily overdo it, so take time to carefully plan your next meal.

It's not a lack of willpower—sugar is highly addictive.

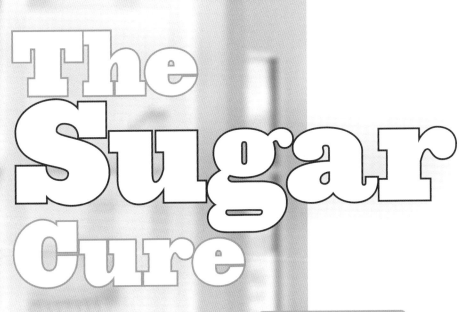

The Sugar Cure

FOR MANY PEOPLE, THE FIRST HURDLE ON A DETOX IS DISENGAGING FROM A SWEETS HABIT—BUT IT'S THE KEY TO GETTING YOUR SYSTEM BACK IN ORDER.

The simplest way to detox? Go off sugar. There's a reason that cutting out added sugars is No. 1 on many cleanse lists: Sugar has a lot to answer for. There was a time when researchers felt that fat was the greatest health risk, because of its effect on cholesterol, and even counseled that while sugar might be bad for your teeth and was empty calories, that was the extent of its danger. That has now been soundly debunked by reams of research that show sugar's toxic role in inflammation, Type 2 diabetes, heart disease, cancer and obesity, to name just a few ailments.

"Sugar, along with processed foods, is thought to be at the root of today's public health crises," says Gavin Van De Walle, MS, RD, president of Dakota Dietitians. Not only has high consumption of sugary foods been linked to the above roster of chronic diseases, says Van De Walle, but "these diseases hinder your body's ability to naturally detoxify itself by harming organs that play an important role, such as your liver and kidneys. For example, high consumption of sugary beverages can cause fatty liver, a condition that negatively impacts liver function." And if your No.1 detoxing organ is operating at a reduced capacity, other toxins beyond sugar are being allowed to circulate through your system and cause damage.

"Sugar's not dangerous because of its calories, or because it makes you fat," wrote Robert Lustig, MD, MSL, professor emeritus of pediatric endocrinology at the University of California, San Francisco, in his landmark essay, "The Toxic Truth About Sugar." "Sugar is dangerous because it's sugar. It's not nutrition. When consumed in excess, it's a toxin. And it's addictive." Lustig has expanded the list of conditions caused by too much sugar to also include suppressed immune system, hyperactivity, inability to concentrate, anxiety, depression, ADD/ADHD, premature aging, arthritis, headaches, overeating,

mood swings, asthma and allergies, highly acidic blood and insomnia. Here's how you can flush sugar out of your system—for good.

Why It's Hard to Quit

People have been beating up on themselves for their sweet tooth for decades, but research has shown that, at least for some people, it is powerfully addictive. Brain scan studies have shown how fructose (a form of sugar used extensively in processed foods) affects the dopamine system, which controls the experience of pleasure. Consuming lots of added sugar changes the brain in ways that look similar to changes in the brains of people addicted to alcohol or to drugs such as cocaine. Yes, there is a real "sugar high," and it puts you on a roller coaster that starts in your brain and affects your whole body.

A study in the journal *Neuroscience* found that, in rats, there was a "neurochemical similarity between intermittent bingeing on sucrose [another form of refined sugar] and drugs of abuse." Another study, in the journal *Nutrients*, showed that high levels of fructose may lead to "neurobiological and physiological alterations

NOT SWEET
"SUGAR TURNS ON THE AGING PROGRAMS IN YOUR BODY," SAYS ROBERT LUSTIG, MD. "THE MORE SUGAR YOU EAT, THE FASTER YOU AGE."

associated with addictive and metabolic disorders." And a review in the *British Journal of Sports Medicine* titled "Sugar Addiction: Is It Real?" answered that question with a resounding yes. Sugar hijacks your pleasure centers in the way addictive drugs do, inducing bingeing, craving and tolerance; and when you suddenly stop taking it in, you can literally have withdrawal symptoms, as you would from an opioid.

But there's another reason why it's hard to "just quit" a sugar habit: It's everywhere, even where you don't expect. This includes savory foods such as sauces, condiments, soups and many other processed foods people don't consider sweet. A study in the journal *BMJ Open* looked at "ultra-processed foods" (those "industrial formulations" full of salt, sugar, oils, fats and flavor additives that result in a label full of unpronounceable ingredients) and found two shocking facts: These foods comprise nearly 60% of the standard American diet, and the content of added sugars in such foods is five times higher than in unprocessed or minimally processed foods. Their conclusion was that ultra-processed foods contribute almost 90% of the added sugars eaten in the United States.

If you're not clued in to this, you may not be cutting sugar even when you think you are by nixing obvious culprits such as cookies

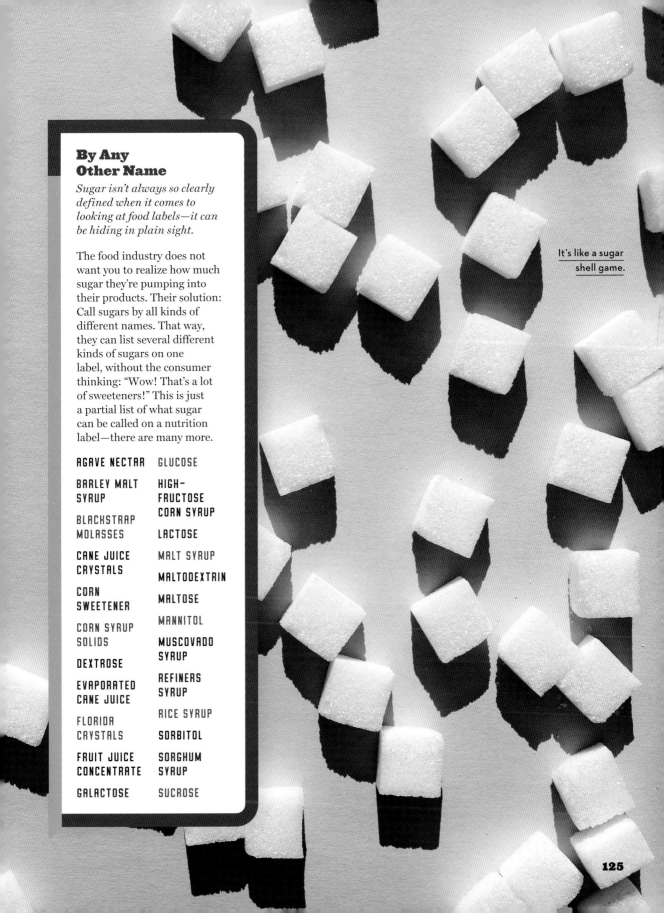

By Any Other Name

Sugar isn't always so clearly defined when it comes to looking at food labels—it can be hiding in plain sight.

The food industry does not want you to realize how much sugar they're pumping into their products. Their solution: Call sugars by all kinds of different names. That way, they can list several different kinds of sugars on one label, without the consumer thinking: "Wow! That's a lot of sweeteners!" This is just a partial list of what sugar can be called on a nutrition label—there are many more.

AGAVE NECTAR	GLUCOSE
BARLEY MALT SYRUP	HIGH-FRUCTOSE CORN SYRUP
BLACKSTRAP MOLASSES	LACTOSE
CANE JUICE CRYSTALS	MALT SYRUP
CORN SWEETENER	MALTODEXTRIN
	MALTOSE
CORN SYRUP SOLIDS	MANNITOL
DEXTROSE	MUSCOVADO SYRUP
EVAPORATED CANE JUICE	REFINERS SYRUP
FLORIDA CRYSTALS	RICE SYRUP
	SORBITOL
FRUIT JUICE CONCENTRATE	SORGHUM SYRUP
GALACTOSE	SUCROSE

It's like a sugar shell game.

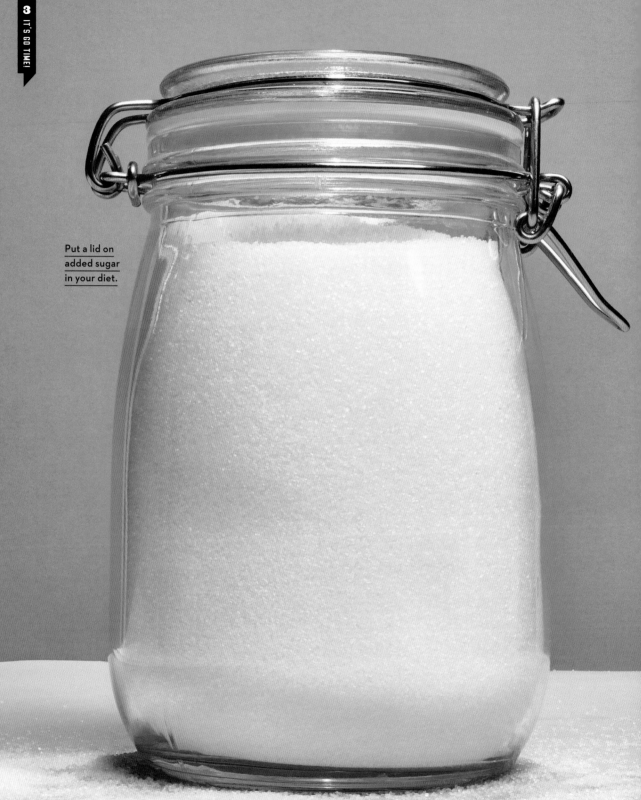

Put a lid on
added sugar
in your diet.

and soft drinks. And as long as you're taking in these hidden sugars, your dopamine centers are being triggered again and again in a vicious cycle. To break that, try the following strategies.

Take It Slow

For one thing, if you've become sugar-dependent, you'll trigger more intense cravings by quitting all at once. And there may be a psychological price as well, because trying to cut "all sugar" can create stress, turning on your fight-or-flight mechanisms and increasing hormones such as cortisol that, in turn, raise blood sugar levels—in essence

That sugar *buzz* carries a high price.

defeating the purpose. There is also evidence that you can retrain your tastes over time, as your brain weans itself from the sugar highs. "Try to consume foods in their natural, unsweetened state," advises Franziska Spritzler, RD, a certified diabetes educator. "Learn to appreciate the sweetness of fruit and the subtle flavors of nuts and other whole foods." The flavors will become more apparent as you cut down on supersweet foods.

Don't Worry About Whole-Food Sugars

Speaking of eating fruit: Go right ahead. The natural sugars in foods such as fresh strawberries, watermelon or apples are different from the added sweeteners that are being pumped into processed foods. Fruit contains glucose, fructose and a combination of the two called sucrose, in far smaller amounts than packaged foods do. It also has fiber, which slows the release of sugar into your

blood, and other nutrients such as vitamins and antioxidants. All this means that natural sugars enter your system slowly, without causing the sugar spikes (and dopamine hit) of concentrated sugars. There are two forms of fruit, though, that aren't a good idea: dried fruit (it has much more sugar than whole fruit) and fruit juices, which are concentrated and lack all fiber. Go for the whole thing—peel and all, if possible.

DAMAGE ABOUT A THIRD OF AMERICAN ADULTS HAVE NONALCOHOLIC FATTY LIVER DISEASE, WHICH IS LINKED TO EXCESS SUGAR CONSUMPTION.

Cut Processed Foods

You'll want to be doing this anyway as part of any cleanse or detox. But eliminating all packaged foods is the No. 1 way to instantly lower your sugar intake. The multiple sugars used by the food industry differ in nature and structure from whole-food sugars, and they're used in huge amounts to boost flavor. If you do buy something in a package, become a good label-reader; sugars go by many stealth names. (See sidebar, page 125.)

Be Careful at Night

You're not imagining it: You do get more cravings at night, for both sugary snacks and salty ones. A study in the journal *Obesity* found that the body's circadian clock increases hunger for sweet, starchy and salty foods in the evening. Researchers hypothesize that consuming more at night may have helped our ancestors store energy to survive times of food scarcity. Have a cup of herbal tea instead.

Hang in There

Lustig feels it takes three weeks of no added sugar to normalize your brain's dopamine system. That also gives your taste buds time to adjust to more subtle sweetness than that offered by the food industry.

Should *You* Get
Juiced?

JUICE CLEANSES ARE BOTH THE MOST POPULAR AND THE MOST CONTROVERSIAL
OF DETOX TECHNIQUES. READ THIS BEFORE YOU SIGN ON.

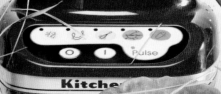

Kitche

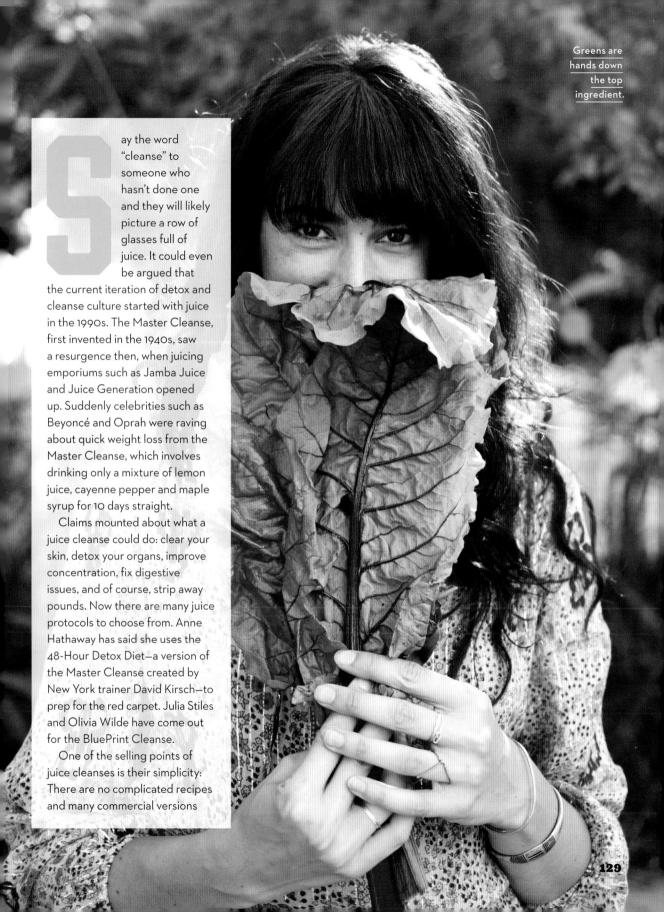

Say the word "cleanse" to someone who hasn't done one and they will likely picture a row of glasses full of juice. It could even be argued that the current iteration of detox and cleanse culture started with juice in the 1990s. The Master Cleanse, first invented in the 1940s, saw a resurgence then, when juicing emporiums such as Jamba Juice and Juice Generation opened up. Suddenly celebrities such as Beyoncé and Oprah were raving about quick weight loss from the Master Cleanse, which involves drinking only a mixture of lemon juice, cayenne pepper and maple syrup for 10 days straight.

Claims mounted about what a juice cleanse could do: clear your skin, detox your organs, improve concentration, fix digestive issues, and of course, strip away pounds. Now there are many juice protocols to choose from. Anne Hathaway has said she uses the 48-Hour Detox Diet—a version of the Master Cleanse created by New York trainer David Kirsch—to prep for the red carpet. Julia Stiles and Olivia Wilde have come out for the BluePrint Cleanse.

One of the selling points of juice cleanses is their simplicity: There are no complicated recipes and many commercial versions supply you with bottles of the elixirs. Another point is their speed; after all, if you go on a liquid diet for three days or more, you're likely to drop pounds quickly. But are they wise? "Fresh juices contain lots of essential vitamins, minerals and antioxidants," says Ansley Hill, RDN, LD, a registered dietitian in Portland, Oregon. "Many people find juicing to be a simple and delicious way to boost their intake of these." But, she adds: "All of the possible benefits of a juice cleanse can be achieved by eating more whole fruits and vegetables—with the added bonus of fiber." Here are the pros and cons of juice cleanses.

The Science Behind It

There's not much research that has examined juice cleanses. But one study published in the journal *Scientific Reports* showed some promising results. When participants drank six bottles a day of fruit-and-vegetable juice blends for three days, they had a "significant decrease" in body weight, and the weight stayed off over the next two weeks. The reason for that might lie in the other result researchers found: The three-day juice diet "induced significant changes in the intestinal microbiota." The two most common types of gut bacteria in humans are *Firmicutes*,

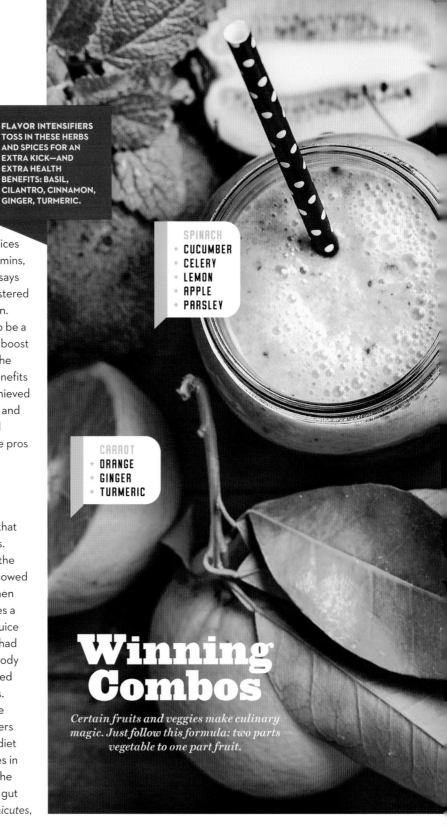

FLAVOR INTENSIFIERS
TOSS IN THESE HERBS AND SPICES FOR AN EXTRA KICK—AND EXTRA HEALTH BENEFITS: BASIL, CILANTRO, CINNAMON, GINGER, TURMERIC.

SPINACH
+ CUCUMBER
+ CELERY
+ LEMON
+ APPLE
+ PARSLEY

CARROT
+ ORANGE
+ GINGER
+ TURMERIC

Winning Combos

Certain fruits and veggies make culinary magic. Just follow this formula: two parts vegetable to one part fruit.

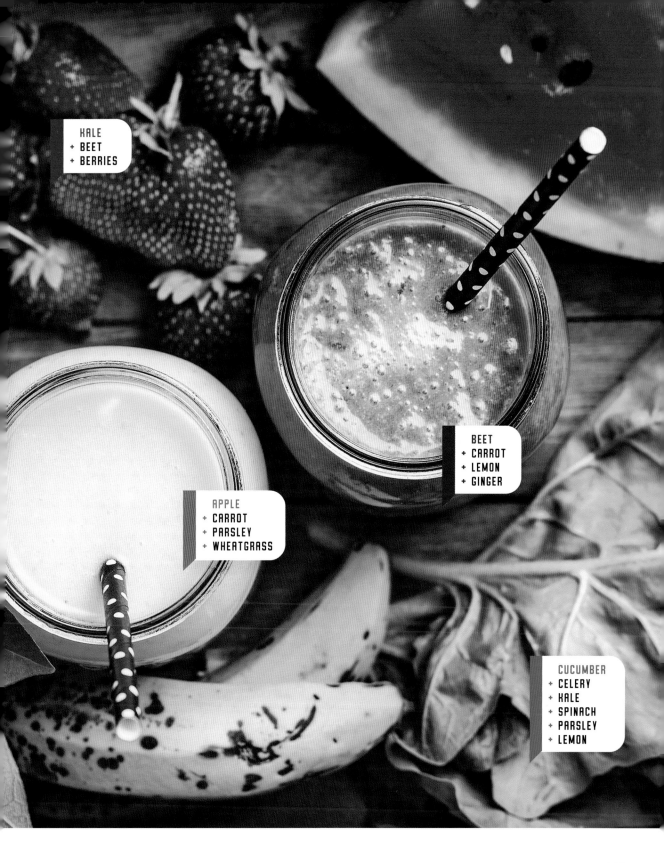

KALE
+ BEET
+ BERRIES

BEET
+ CARROT
+ LEMON
+ GINGER

APPLE
+ CARROT
+ PARSLEY
+ WHEATGRASS

CUCUMBER
+ CELERY
+ KALE
+ SPINACH
+ PARSLEY
+ LEMON

linked to increased body weight, and *Bacteroidetes*, linked to low body weight. After the juicing, the number of *Firmicutes* dropped, while *Bacteroidetes* increased significantly, potentially setting up people for weight loss.

Specific juices also may have particular benefits. One study of people with high cholesterol found that drinking 5 ounces of kale juice daily for three months reduced LDL (bad) cholesterol by 10% and boosted heart-protective HDL cholesterol by 27%. Other studies show that citrus-based juices and carrot juice may reduce heart-disease risk, and that carrot juice may reduce oxidative stress in cells in women treated for breast cancer. But the Harvard T.H. Chan School of Public Health points out that while certain juices are linked to health benefits, drinking a glass of kale juice every day is a far cry from a juice cleanse. "No published research currently supports the safety or efficacy of juice cleanses or fasts," according to Harvard researchers.

Ups and Downs

Why are juice cleanses so popular? Here's how it boils down. **Pros** There's no question that fruits and vegetables are loaded with vitamins, minerals and plant compounds known to reduce inflammation, prevent disease and promote overall health. "Research shows that drinking fruit and vegetable juice could be an

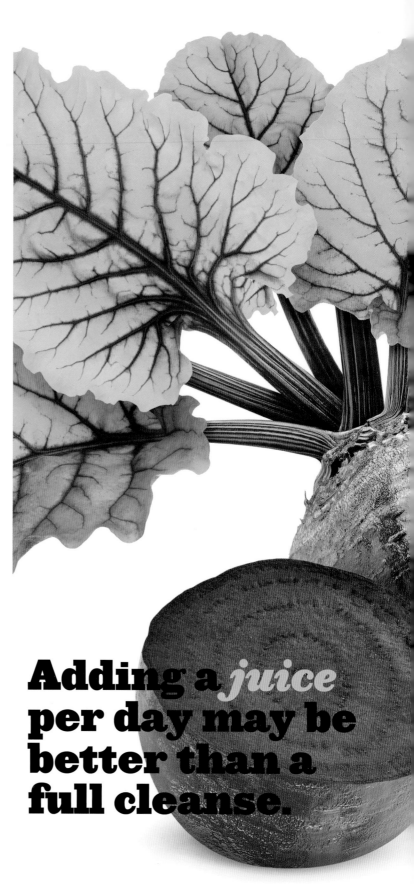

Adding a *juice* per day may be better than a full cleanse.

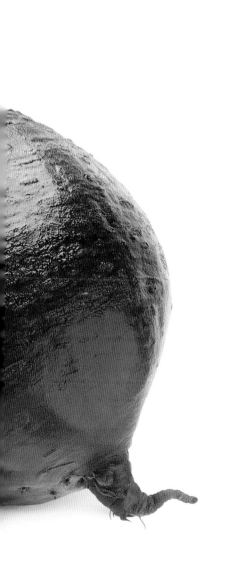

efficient way to access these benefits," says Hill. Juice may also help the microbiome, she adds. "Many fruit and vegetable juices contain nutrients that function as prebiotics, the carbohydrates that feed the healthy bacteria in your gut and promote digestive health." But the benefits of juicing are similar to those you would get by simply eating more whole fruits and veggies. "For some people, it may be easier to drink these nutrient-rich foods than to prepare full meals centered around them," she says.

Cons There are drawbacks to juicing, especially for extended periods of time. Most juices are high in sugar (especially those made from fruits), and studies have found that one extra serving per day of juice may be associated with a higher risk of Type 2 diabetes in women. Juices also lack nutrients such as fiber and protein—both of which increase satiation longer and help stabilize blood glucose spikes from natural sugars in juice. "Eating whole fruit, not just juice, lends itself to a slower, more manageable rise in blood sugar, partly because consuming it takes longer," says Hill. "Also, it's a lot easier to accidentally overconsume calories and sugar from juice than from whole foods." Some people also have headaches and fatigue on a juice cleanse. While proponents claim these are

signs your body is detoxing, many dietitians feel these side effects are due to fluctuating blood sugar and a lack of protein.

Juice Rules

How can you get the best out of juicing while avoiding the hazards? Follow these guidelines:

The 3-Day Rule If you do a full-on, juice-only cleanse, limit it to three days. Evidence shows few risks of a short-term juice fast.

Do It Part Time Certain juices do have special benefits, so it's not a bad idea to work in one juice a day to cover your nutritional bases. "If you find it hard to meet the daily recommendations for fruits and vegetables, juicing may be a viable option," says Hill. "Just make sure that juice doesn't make you consume more calories than you need."

Consider Smoothies Smoothies are blended rather than pressed, so they retain the food's fiber. Also, you can add a healthy fat (such as avocado or nut butter) and/or protein powder, which makes the drink a complete meal.

Choose Your Produce Well There's a world of difference, nutritionally, between a mostly fruit drink and one that's mostly vegetables—especially if the veggies are superfoods such as kale, beets, spinach, carrots, wheatgrass, parsley and celery.

Make Your Own Not only are store-bought juices expensive, but many of them can quickly oxidize and lose their benefits.

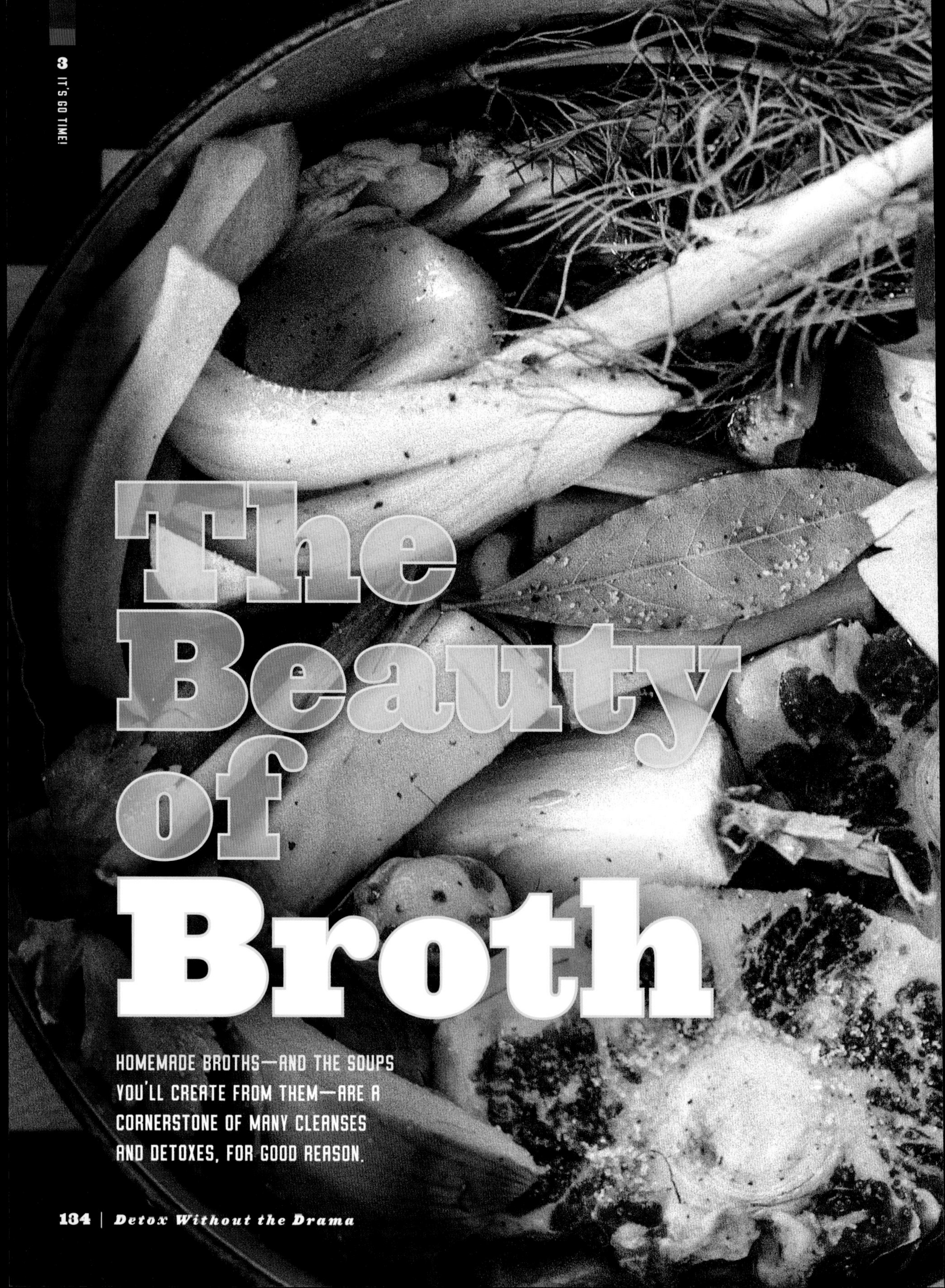

The Beauty of Broth

HOMEMADE BROTHS—AND THE SOUPS
YOU'LL CREATE FROM THEM—ARE A
CORNERSTONE OF MANY CLEANSES
AND DETOXES, FOR GOOD REASON.

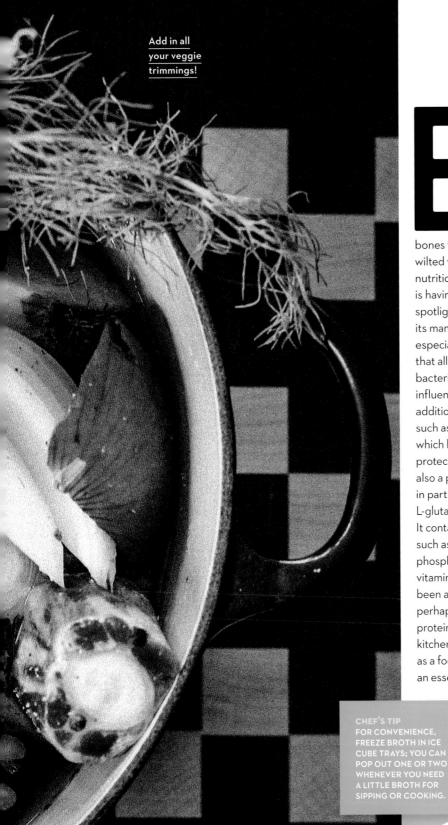

Add in all
your veggie
trimmings!

Broth made from bones, vegetables or a combination of the two is a time-honored foodstuff, central to almost every cuisine and culture. It's thrifty (you can even use bones from a cooked chicken, or wilted veggies), and it's outrageously nutritious. But this ancient recipe is having a new moment in the spotlight, as science has pinpointed its many additional benefits—especially for the microbiome, that all-important colony of helpful bacteria that lives in your gut and influences your immune system. In addition, broth contains nutrients such as collagen and cartilage, which help repair sore muscles and protect joints from stress. Broth is also a powerful anti-inflammatory, in part due to an amino acid called L-glutamine. Need more proof? It contains vitamins and nutrients such as calcium, magnesium, phosphorous, iron, selenium, and vitamins A and K. Plus, broth has been associated with weight loss, perhaps because it's high in satiating protein and low in calories. In your kitchen, broth functions not only as a food unto itself, but also as an essential ingredient in all kinds of hearty cleansing soups that form the basis for many a healthy dinner. To make it yourself, see the Chicken Bone Broth recipe on page 162.

CHEF'S TIP
FOR CONVENIENCE, FREEZE BROTH IN ICE CUBE TRAYS; YOU CAN POP OUT ONE OR TWO WHENEVER YOU NEED A LITTLE BROTH FOR SIPPING OR COOKING.

Boo

St Your Cleanse

CERTAIN SUPPLEMENTS CAN HELP USHER OUT TOXINS, REDUCE INFLAMMATION AND SUPPORT KEY ORGANS—BUT CHOOSE WISELY.

Don't overdo it! You'll need only a few essentials.

The world of supplements is a thicket—as you may have noticed in a trip down the vitamin aisle of your local drugstore. It's also an expensive landscape, and it's possible to spend a small fortune if you're not careful. There are currently more than 90,000 supplements on the market, and Americans shell out more than $32 billion a year to buy them.

Once you decide to do a detox or cleanse, things can get even more costly. Many commercial cleanses put packets of supplements front and center,

biochemistry explains why some of these traditional remedies were, and still are, effective. Bennett's solution: "Take the best of both the old and the new."

Particular supplements may aid your body during a cleanse, but there are also some that are capable of causing harm if misused or taken in large doses. For example, take antioxidant supplements, such as beta-carotene or vitamin A. "These are popular and commonly considered healthy," says Gavin Van De Walle, MS, RD, owner of

supplements in high amounts can do just the opposite." Studies have shown that antioxidants did not lower cancer risk, and several meta-analyses have found that supplements of beta-carotene (a precursor of vitamin A) actually increased the risk of bladder cancer (and, in smokers, of lung cancer as well). Vitamin A itself can increase the risk of birth defects in pregnant women taking high doses.

The safest road is the middle one: Remember that "the devil is in the dose," and many of the

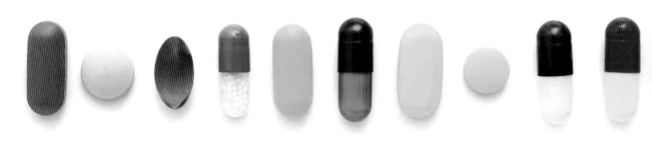

promising magical results. That's a powerful message to those who would like a shortcut to health, a silver bullet that does all the work while you sit back and wait. That's not the answer, but neither is throwing out the baby with the bathwater, says Peter Bennett, ND, co-author of *7-Day Detox Miracle*. "For thousands of years, herbs, clays and special substances have been used to assist in purifying the body and supporting it during detoxification—especially those that stimulated and protected the liver," Bennett says. Now

Dakota Dietitians. "That's partly because fruits and vegetables, which are rich in antioxidants, are associated with many health benefits, including a reduced risk of disease."

Once you isolate and concentrate certain substances, however, the health equation can change. "It's commonly thought that taking antioxidant supplements prevents the damage caused by free radicals to the body's cells, helping to ward off disease and promote longevity," Van De Walle explains. "But taking antioxidant

cleansing benefits claimed by supplement makers are just as powerful, if not more so, when you take in vitamins, minerals, amino acids and antioxidants from your food. That said, certain supplements, in moderation, may speed your detoxification progress. These four comprise a good baseline.

1 Vitamin C

"Vitamin C is critical in the assembly of connective tissue that surrounds cells, and a deficiency causes the extracellular matrix to

For Your Consideration

Looking for an extra boost? Add these cleansing supplements to the Big Four:

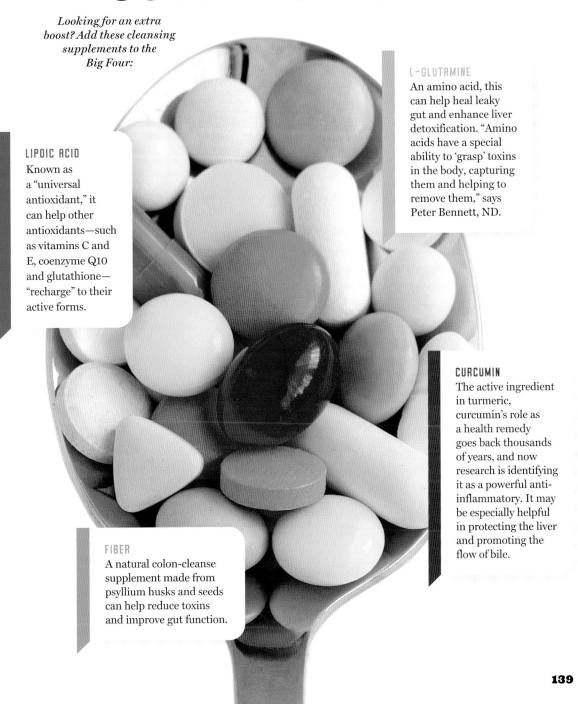

LIPOIC ACID
Known as a "universal antioxidant," it can help other antioxidants—such as vitamins C and E, coenzyme Q10 and glutathione— "recharge" to their active forms.

L-GLUTAMINE
An amino acid, this can help heal leaky gut and enhance liver detoxification. "Amino acids have a special ability to 'grasp' toxins in the body, capturing them and helping to remove them," says Peter Bennett, ND.

CURCUMIN
The active ingredient in turmeric, curcumin's role as a health remedy goes back thousands of years, and now research is identifying it as a powerful anti-inflammatory. It may be especially helpful in protecting the liver and promoting the flow of bile.

FIBER
A natural colon-cleanse supplement made from psyllium husks and seeds can help reduce toxins and improve gut function.

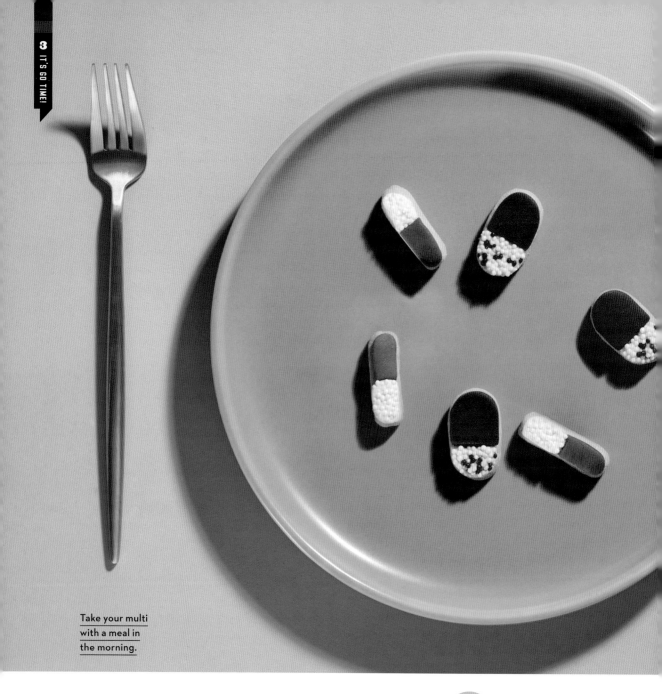

Take your multi
with a meal in
the morning.

become weak and fragile," says
Bennett. That's especially key
with intestinal cells, as leaky gut
syndrome can lead to toxins
seeping out into surrounding
tissue. "Vitamin C appears to
be a kind of universal antitoxin,"
Bennett says. In the clinic he ran

in Langley, British Columbia,
Canada, it was regarded as "the
most important supplement for
detoxification." Vitamin C helps
detox the liver, and is water-
soluble. So, unlike with vitamin A,
any excess your body can't use is
simply excreted.

2 A Multi-vitamin

Although many
experts feel that a full-spectrum
supplement is not necessary if
you eat a well-rounded diet, there
is also no harm in taking one—and
during a cleanse, when you are

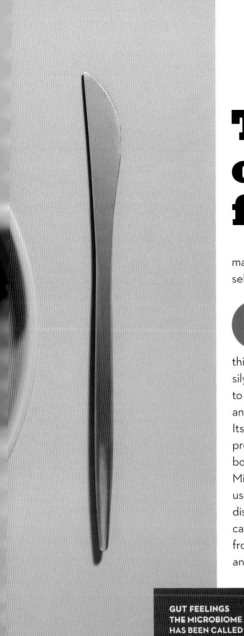

Try to get most of your *benefits* from food.

manganese, molybdenum, selenium and magnesium.

③ Milk Thistle
This herbal remedy, derived from the milk thistle plant, has high levels of silymarin, which has been shown to have antioxidant, anti-viral and anti-inflammatory properties. Its biggest benefit, though, is its protective effect on the liver—the body's primary cleansing organ. Milk thistle has traditionally been used to treat liver and gallbladder disorders, prevent and treat cancer, and even protect the liver from snakebite venom, alcohol and other environmental toxins.

Studies have shown improvement in liver function in those with liver disease who took a milk thistle supplement; researchers hypothesize that it reduces damage to the liver caused by free radicals, which are produced when your liver metabolizes toxic substances.

Milk thistle has also been used as a traditional remedy for neurological conditions such as dementia, and in test tube and animal studies silymarin has been shown to prevent oxidative damage to brain cells. Its other benefits—including improving acne and possibly aiding in cancer treatment—are likely due to its powerful anti-inflammatory effects. Bennett calls milk thistle a "wonder plant." Consult with your doctor before adding to your daily regimen.

④ Probiotics
One goal of cleanses or detox programs is to improve the bacterial status of your gut microbiome, which research increasingly shows is essential to your overall health. You can have a powerful effect on your gut bacteria through diet alone, but during a cleanse it's a good idea to "reseed" your bacteria by taking a probiotic, says Bennett. "This creates an optimum, balanced environment, protecting the intestines and the rest of the body from dangerous bacterial insurgents," he explains. He advises looking for *Lactobacillus acidophilus* and *L. bifidus* strains among the many types that are available at the drugstore.

GUT FEELINGS
THE MICROBIOME HAS BEEN CALLED THE "SECOND BRAIN" BECAUSE IT HAS BEEN IMPLICATED IN CONDITIONS SUCH AS DEPRESSION.

changing up your diet, it can ensure a baseline intake of vitamins and minerals. Bennett advises looking for one that contains at least the recommended daily allowances of vitamins A, B-complex and E, along with zinc, copper,

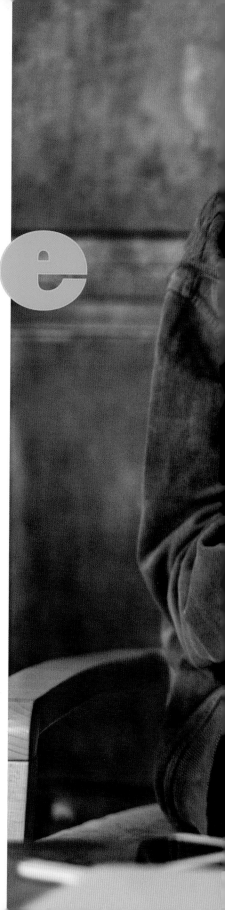

The Write Stuff

KEEPING A JOURNAL AT THE START OF A CLEANSE OR
DETOX CAN HELP YOU BECOME MORE FULLY AWARE OF
WHAT YOU HOPE TO GAIN FROM THE PROCESS.

There's something very powerful about a pen and a blank piece of paper. Writing down your thoughts, fears, hopes, aspirations, memories and goals makes everything seem a little less abstract and a little more concrete. And when you are kicking off a detox program or cleanse, maintaining a journal can help you become more fully aware of your intentions—and what you truly hope to gain from the process beyond the physical changes taking place.

"Journaling is an ideal way to build self-awareness and become more in tune with what you are feeling," notes Sara Robinson, author of *Choose You: A Guided Self-Care Journal Made Just for You!* and a mental-skills coach. "It helps make a connection between your thoughts and actions."

Research has long backed the concept of journaling as a way to clear your mind and face whatever emotional challenges you may be dealing with, from reducing stress, anxiety and depression to helping you sort through goals and establish a sense of meaning and purpose. "There is a great deal of information out there regarding the power of journaling,"

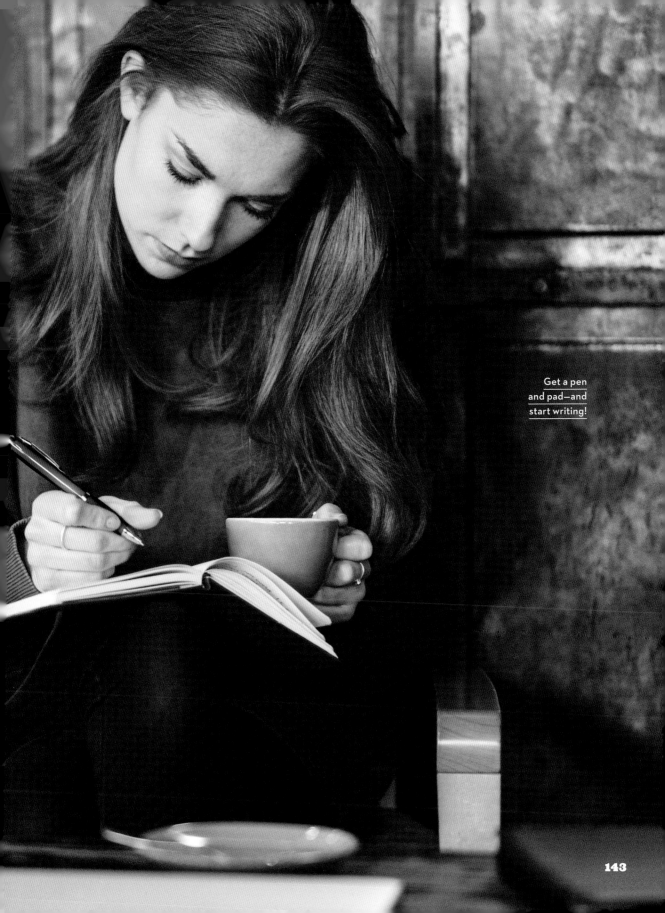

Get a pen
and pad—and
start writing!

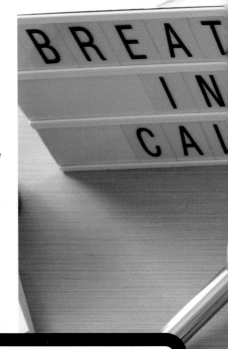

notes Lisa M. Schab, LCSW, a psychotherapist based in Libertyville, Illinois, and the author of 25 self-help books, including the upcoming *Put Your Worries Here: A Creative Journal for Teens With Anxiety.* "There's an incredibly strong mind-body connection that takes place with writing down your thoughts."

Of course, you don't have to be doing a special detox or cleanse to keep a journal, but it's a good time to start. "It's a great way to record your experiences and remember them—the positives as well as the negatives—so you have a standing record of what went on," says Robinson. "It helps you see the changes you've made and gives you a sense of how far you may have come."

The act of writing something down also makes it seem more real, whether that's putting down a goal you want to reach

7 Ways to Make Journaling Easier

Got writer's block? Try using some of these simple strategies to help get your thoughts (and your pen) moving.

1 FIND A TIME THAT WORKS
The more often you journal, the easier it gets. Keeping a regular writing time (morning, afternoon, evening) helps you form a habit. Try doing it with your morning coffee or before bed at night. Having a regular place to sit—a cozy corner, a comfy couch—can also help you keep it up.

2 TAKE IT SLOW
You don't have to fill out every page of a notebook. "You could spend a half hour or more writing, but that can feel like a lot. You really only need a few minutes to put your thoughts and experiences on paper," says mental-skills coach Sara Robinson. Even two minutes of writing can make a difference.

3 LET GO
If you are in a zone, don't cut yourself off too soon. "To me, the best journaling takes place when you get lost in it," says therapist Lisa Schab. "Don't think too much—let the words flow."

4 DON'T SWEAT THE GRAMMAR
Or punctuation. You can use bullet points, brief sentences, phrases—whatever it takes to get the words down. No one will be spell-checking or editing this, so don't worry about how it reads or sounds.

5 REREAD IT (IF YOU WANT)
Much of the process of journaling is about putting the words down. But it can also be helpful to read over them at a later time, says Robinson. "Consider checking back after a few weeks or months and reflecting on what you've written," she adds. "It can help deepen your understanding of a situation once you've had some perspective."

6 USE PROMPTS
"Prompts are a good way to help you get rolling," says Schab. Find some at the end of this section on page 147. Need more? Just spitball—there are really no limits to what you can write about.

7 THINK OUTSIDE THE PEN
You can journal the old-fashioned way (in a notebook), but if you'd rather journal on a computer or other device, that works too! You can even keep an audio journal, using voice memos on a phone or some other recording device.

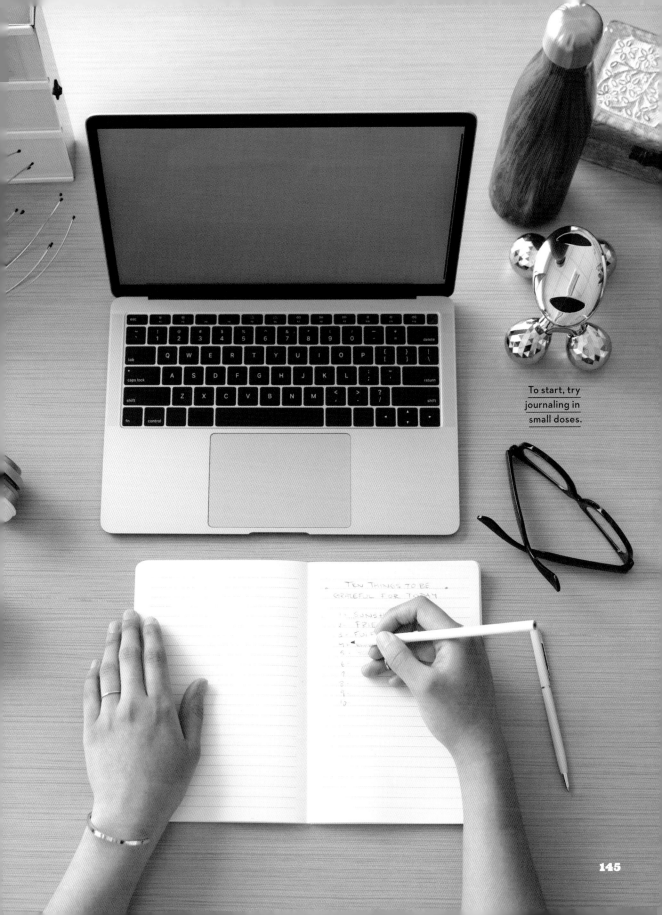

To start, try journaling in small doses.

Take time
to write down
your goals.

after you've finished your reset plan, or helping you deal with a problem in your work or personal life. "Taking those thoughts and feelings that are internal and making them external by writing them down makes them seem more real and allows you to take ownership," adds Robinson.

When Words Surprise

Many journal keepers are surprised at what comes through the other end of the pen. "When something comes down from deep inside you and you don't stop to judge, critique or analyze it, you may not have even realized you were thinking that way," says Schab. "You may experience emotional revelations that are similar to talk therapy."

You may also be amazed at how much you enjoy spending time with your journal. "A lot of people think they have to be a good writer to keep a journal, but often they'll discover how fun and easy it is," says Robinson.

And when you journal on a regular basis, she adds, you'll likely find yourself being more mindful in other situations. "Often, you are able to consider a situation and your reaction to it without getting overly emotional about it."

Getting Started

Rule No. 1 of journaling: There are no rules. "People are often worried that they'll do something wrong, but there's really no 'wrong way' to keep a journal," says Schab. "It's simply a matter of setting aside some time and starting to write."

If you need some prompts to help you kick things off, consider some thought-provoking prompts, such as listing what makes you feel grateful, goals you want to set or reach, what has challenged you the most, what you want to gain from your cleanse or detox, and how you are feeling before, during and after.

Surprising Health Benefits

We know keeping a journal can help you feel better, and there's scientific evidence it can also play an important role in keeping you healthier. Here are a few ways how:

IT RELIEVES STRESS
Writing helps you cope with stress and anxiety. Scientists say it can involve the amygdala (the region of your brain that registers emotions and helps determine whether a situation is dangerous or safe) so you feel safe and secure putting your thoughts on paper.

IT BOOSTS THE IMMUNE SYSTEM
Research from the University of Auckland in New Zealand found HIV/AIDS patients who wrote about their life experiences in four 30-minute sessions had higher CD4 lymphocyte counts (a measure of immune function) than a control group.

IT IMPROVES HEART HEALTH
A study from the University of Arizona found that subjects who kept a journal after going through a divorce not only were able to better process their emotions, but also had a lower heart rate and higher heart rate variability (a sign of heart health).

IT SOLIDIFIES MEMORIES
Writing down your experiences can help you remember them more clearly later on, according to research from the University of Lancaster. Expressive writing can also help reduce intrusive thoughts about negative events, and boost working memory.

IT REDUCES SYMPTOMS OF ASTHMA AND RHEUMATOID ARTHRITIS (RA)
A study of 112 patients with asthma or RA found those who wrote about the most stressful event in their lives showed an improvement in their symptoms, compared to a control group.

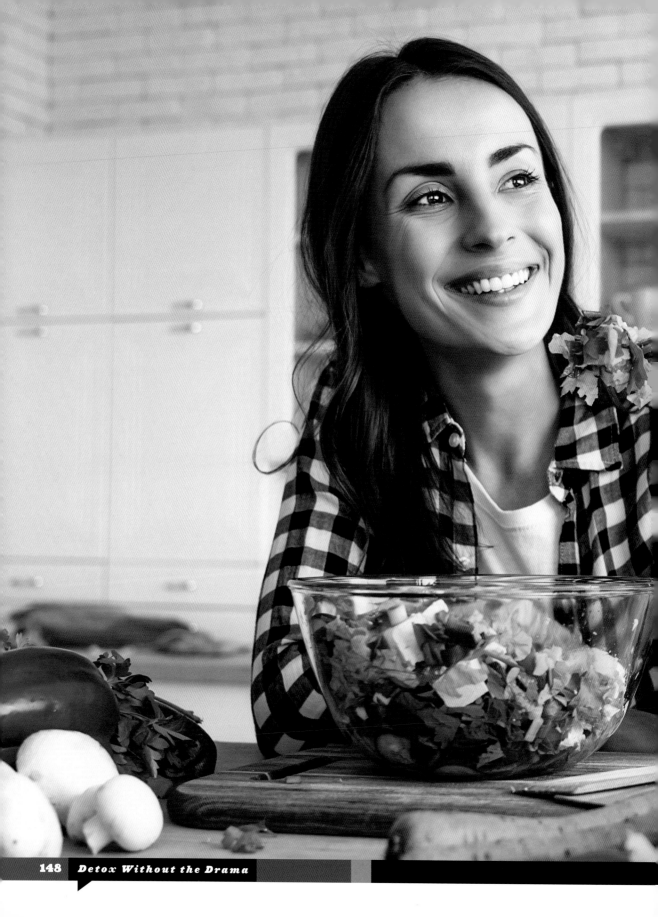

4

HEALTHY RECIPES

YOU DON'T NEED EXPENSIVE PREMADE
MEALS TO RESET YOUR DIET. THESE DELICIOUS
IDEAS ARE CLEAN AND EASY!

Smoothies & Breakfast

FRONT-LOAD YOUR DAY WITH SIMPLE SHAKES AND BOWLS THAT ARE PACKED WITH PHYTONUTRIENTS AND FIBER.

Hearty Smoothie Love

Blend sweet and savory flavors in this antioxidant-packed starter.

START TO FINISH 5 minutes (all active)

SERVINGS 1 (about 16 fluid ounces)

INGREDIENTS

1	cup blueberries
1	heaping handful spinach
¼	avocado, peeled and sliced
1	large banana
1	tablespoon almond butter (optional)
2	cups water or coconut water

INSTRUCTIONS

In a high-speed blender, puree all ingredients until creamy. Pour into a tall glass and enjoy.

TIP
You can sub in peanut butter for the almond butter, but make sure to choose a brand that doesn't have added oils or sugars.

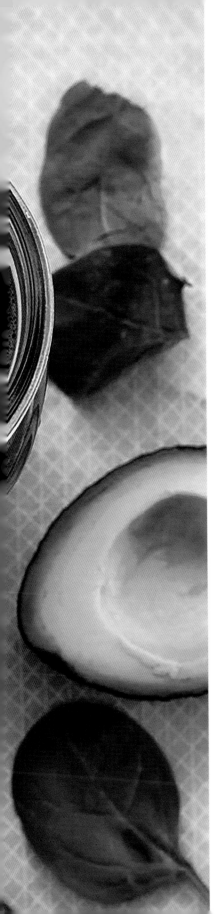

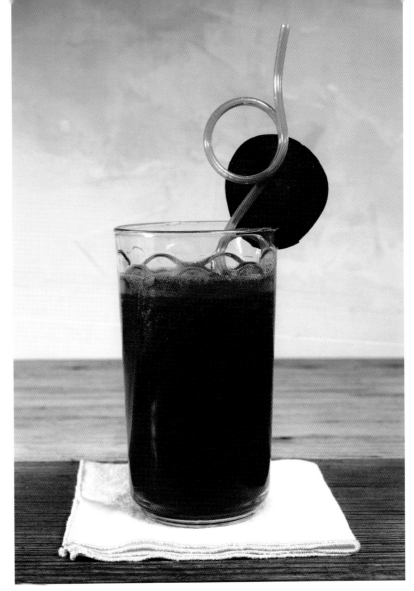

Beet Orange Smoothie

Beets contain high levels of nitrates, which the body converts to nitric oxide to help boost blood flow. This wonderfully sweet blend will make a believer out of even the most beet-averse.

START TO FINISH 5 minutes (all active)
SERVINGS 1 (about 16 fluid ounces)

INGREDIENTS

1½ cups orange juice

1 small beet, peeled and grated
2 mandarin oranges, peeled and separated into segments
GARNISH Beet slice

INSTRUCTIONS

Place ingredients in the blender jar, in the order listed. Blend on low speed for 10 seconds, stopping to scrape down the sides of the jar with a spatula if needed. Blend on high speed for 15 seconds to fully mix. Serve immediately.

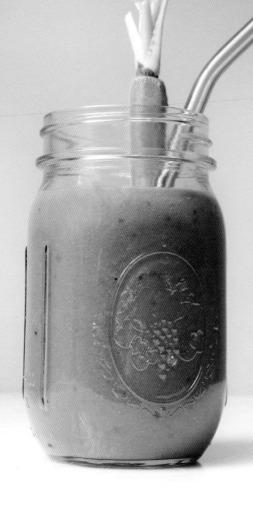

TIP
Pour liquids into the blender first, then powders, grains and other dry ingredients, then leafy greens. Top with heavier solid items.

Carrot Ginger Smoothie

This vitamin-rich smoothie tastes like carrot cake, thanks to ginger, apple and molasses.

START TO FINISH 5 minutes (all active)

SERVINGS 1 (about 16 fluid ounces)

INGREDIENTS

- ½ cup carrot juice
- ½ cup orange juice
- 2 tablespoons sunflower seed butter (can substitute 3 tablespoons roasted sunflower seeds)
- 1 teaspoon molasses
- ½ cup grated carrots
- ½ small apple, cored and chopped
- ½ avocado, peeled and sliced
- 1 teaspoon fresh grated ginger
- GARNISH Baby carrot

INSTRUCTIONS

Place ingredients in the blender jar, in the order listed. Blend on low speed for 10 seconds, stopping to scrape down the sides of the jar with a spatula if needed. Blend on high speed for 15 seconds to fully mix. Serve immediately.

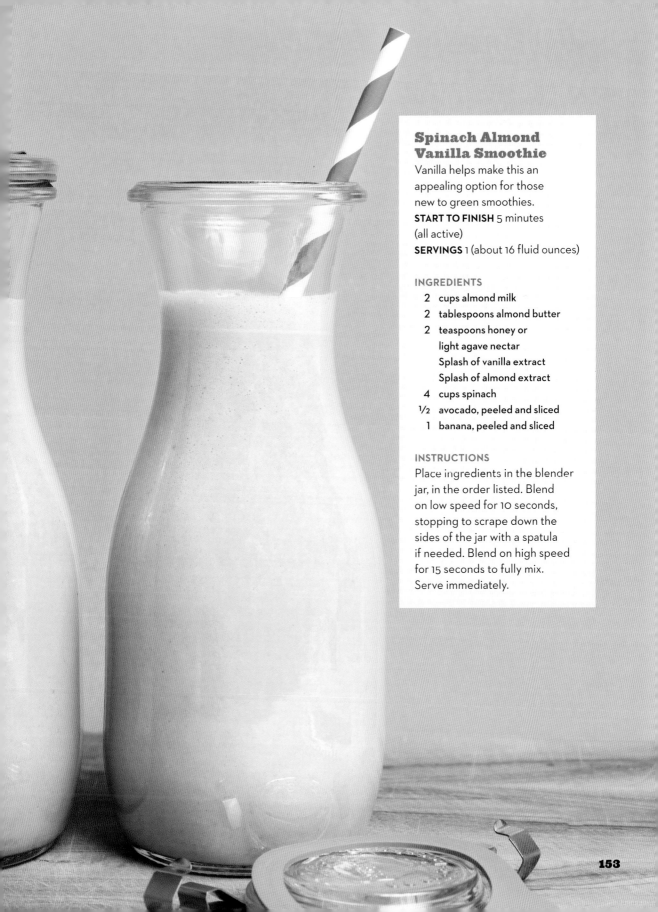

Spinach Almond Vanilla Smoothie

Vanilla helps make this an appealing option for those new to green smoothies.

START TO FINISH 5 minutes (all active)

SERVINGS 1 (about 16 fluid ounces)

INGREDIENTS

2	cups almond milk
2	tablespoons almond butter
2	teaspoons honey or light agave nectar
	Splash of vanilla extract
	Splash of almond extract
4	cups spinach
½	avocado, peeled and sliced
1	banana, peeled and sliced

INSTRUCTIONS

Place ingredients in the blender jar, in the order listed. Blend on low speed for 10 seconds, stopping to scrape down the sides of the jar with a spatula if needed. Blend on high speed for 15 seconds to fully mix. Serve immediately.

Zucchini Cucumber Berry Smoothie

Zucchini gives this blend a creamy texture—and extra nutrition!

START TO FINISH 5 minutes (all active)

SERVINGS 6 (about 8 fluid ounces each)

INGREDIENTS

1½ cups unsweetened almond milk
1 cup applesauce
    Squeeze of lemon juice
2 teaspoons honey or
    light agave nectar
4 tablespoons almond butter
2 cups peeled and
    chopped zucchini
2 cups peeled and
    sliced cucumber
1 cup blueberries
1 cup ice cubes
    GARNISHES Berries, cucumber
    slice

INSTRUCTIONS

Place ingredients in the blender jar, in the order listed. Blend on low speed for 10 seconds, stopping to scrape down the sides of the jar with a spatula if needed. Blend on high speed for 15 seconds to fully mix. Serve immediately.

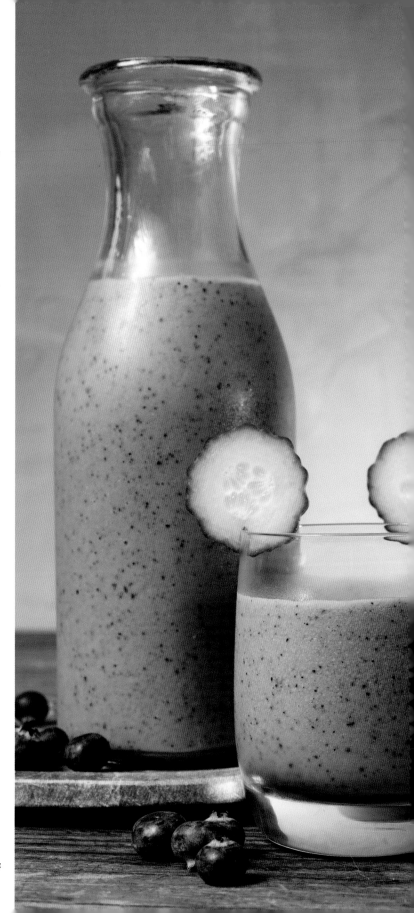

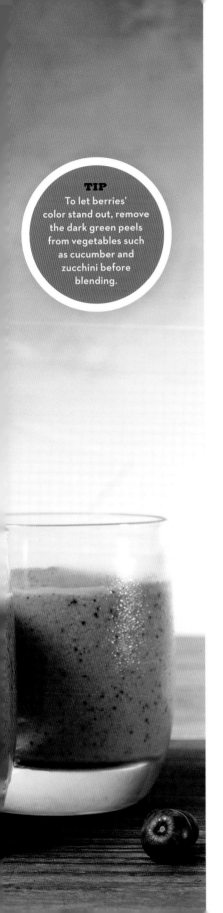

TIP
To let berries' color stand out, remove the dark green peels from vegetables such as cucumber and zucchini before blending.

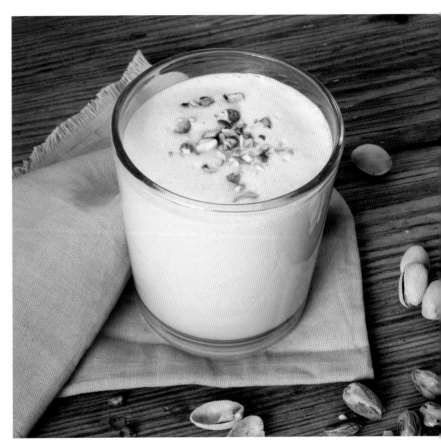

Green Tea Orange Pistachio Smoothie

This combines two sources of antioxidants—green tea and citrus—in one bright and tasty treat to enjoy any time of day.

START TO FINISH 5 minutes (all active)

SERVINGS 1 (about 16 fluid ounces)

INGREDIENTS

- ½ cup strong, brewed and chilled green tea
- ¾ cup unsweetened almond milk
- 1 teaspoon honey or light agave nectar
- 1 mandarin orange, peeled and separated into segments
- ½ small avocado, peeled and diced
- 2 tablespoons chopped pistachios
- GARNISH Chopped pistachios

INSTRUCTIONS

Place ingredients in the blender jar, in the order listed. Blend on low speed for 10 seconds, stopping to scrape down the sides of the jar with a spatula if needed. Blend on high speed for 15 seconds to fully mix. Serve immediately.

Savory Yogurt Bowl With Raw Vegetables

This may not be your typical fruity yogurt bowl, but it's perfect for breakfast or brunch when you want something simple.

START TO FINISH 10 minutes (all active)

SERVINGS 1

INGREDIENTS

- 1 cup Greek yogurt
- 1 scallion, sliced
- 1 small carrot, cut into ribbons
- 1 small Persian cucumber, sliced in half-moons
- 1 large radish, sliced
- 6 cherry tomatoes, halved
- ¼ cup micro parsley greens
- 1 teaspoon black chia seeds

INSTRUCTIONS

1 Place yogurt in a serving bowl.

2 Top with scallion, carrot, cucumber, radish and tomatoes.

3 Sprinkle with micro parsley greens and black chia seeds.

TIP
Fermented, full-fat dairy products—such as Greek yogurt—not only promote the growth of good bacteria in the gut, they also contain lots of vitamin K, which is essential for healthy blood clotting.

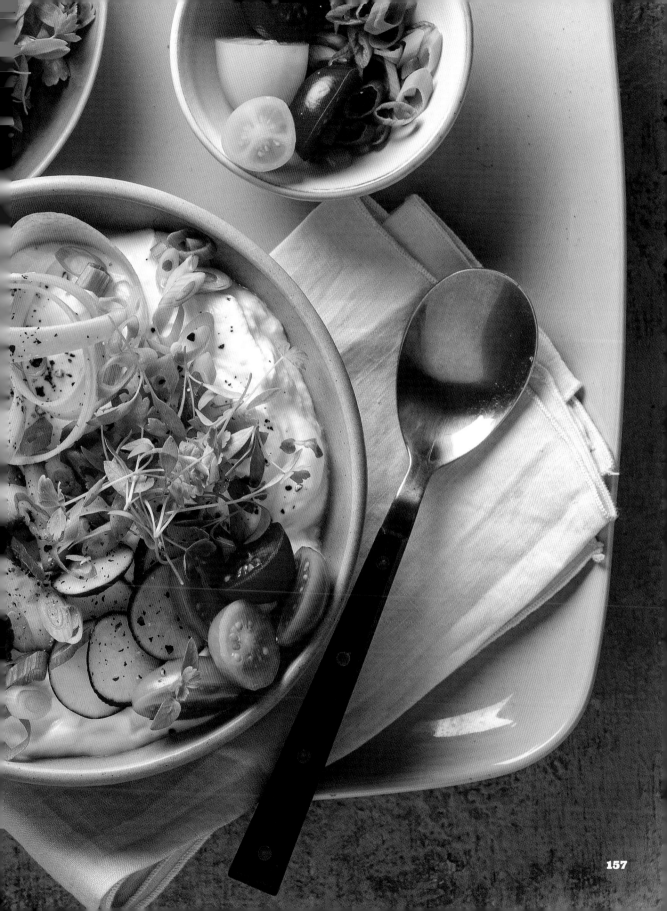

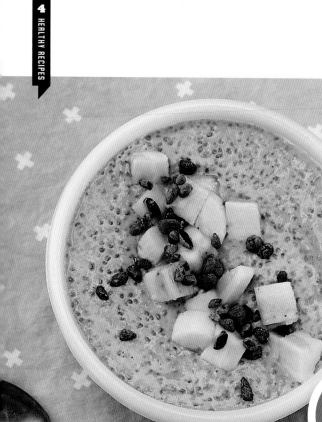

TIP
Hempseeds
and chia seeds
add protein.

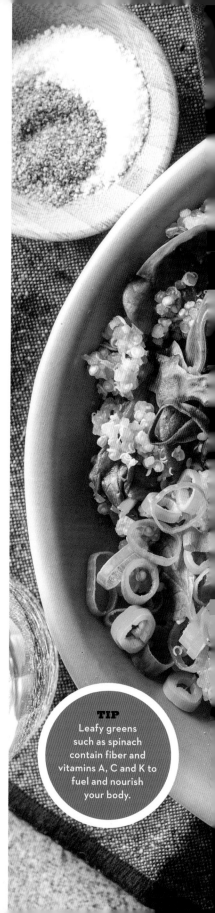

Creamy Banana Chia Pudding

Satisfy a sweet tooth—and your protein needs—with this cereal/pudding hybrid that only feels like it's a cheat on any detox plan.

START TO FINISH 40 minutes (10 minutes active)

SERVINGS 6

INGREDIENTS

- 2 tablespoons hempseeds
- 1 cup water
- 5 dates, pitted
- 2 bananas (plus more, chopped, for garnish, optional)
- ½ teaspoon sea salt
- 1 teaspoon vanilla extract
- 2 tablespoons chia seeds

GARNISHES Banana, cacao nibs, cinnamon

INSTRUCTIONS

1 In a high-speed blender, puree hempseeds and water until completely smooth.

2 Add the dates, bananas, salt and vanilla. Blend until smooth.

3 Pour mixture into a bowl and stir in chia seeds.

4 Let sit for 30 minutes (or, for a super-thick pudding, refrigerate overnight).

5 Top with chopped banana, cacao nibs and/or a sprinkle of cinnamon.

TIP
Leafy greens
such as spinach
contain fiber and
vitamins A, C and K to
fuel and nourish
your body.

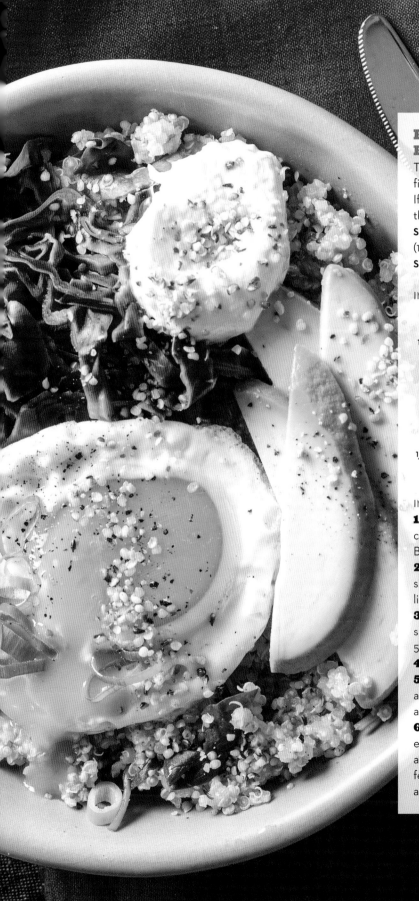

Probiotic Breakfast Bowl

This dish is loaded with protein, fiber, healthy fats and probiotics. If you want to simplify it, take off the fried eggs.

START TO FINISH 30 minutes (10 minutes active)

SERVINGS 4

INGREDIENTS

1	cup uncooked quinoa
2	cups vegetable broth
½	teaspoon sea salt
2	cups baby spinach leaves
4	fried eggs
2	avocados, sliced
3	scallions, sliced
1	cup fermented purple cabbage or kimchi
¼	cup plain Greek yogurt
4	teaspoons hempseeds

INSTRUCTIONS

1 In a medium saucepan, combine quinoa, broth and salt. Bring to a boil.

2 Cover, reduce heat and simmer 15 minutes or until liquid is absorbed.

3 Remove from heat, stir in spinach. Cover and let stand 5 minutes.

4 Meanwhile, fry eggs.

5 Fluff quinoa mixture with a fork and divide evenly among 4 bowls.

6 Top each bowl with a fried egg and equal amounts of avocado slices, scallion slices, fermented cabbage, yogurt and hempseeds.

TIP
Cacao nibs are just
pieces of cocoa beans,
so they're naturally low in
sugar. Sold raw or roasted,
they add magnesium,
copper and fiber to
any dish.

Breakfast Chia Pudding Bowls With Cacao Nibs & Pecans

Make these bowls the night before—so there's no excuse for not having a healthy breakfast!

START TO FINISH 10 minutes (plus overnight)

SERVINGS 2

INGREDIENTS

- ¼ cup chia seeds
- 1 cup almond milk
- 2 teaspoons honey
- 1 teaspoon cacao nibs
- 1 teaspoon chopped pecans

INSTRUCTIONS

1 Between 2 lidded jars, evenly divide chia seeds, almond milk and honey. Cover and shake to mix.

2 Refrigerate overnight.

3 Just before serving, top with cacao nibs and pecans.

Overnight Oats With Blueberries & Walnuts

Creamy and tart like yogurt, but higher in protein and probiotics, kefir is available in both dairy and nondairy versions.

START TO FINISH 5 minutes (plus overnight)

SERVINGS 1

INGREDIENTS

- 1 cup kefir
- ¼ cup gluten-free oats, toasted
- 2 tablespoons black chia seeds
- ½ teaspoon vanilla extract
- 1 tablespoon blueberries
  GARNISHES Walnuts, sunflower seeds

INSTRUCTIONS

1 In a 1-pint Mason jar, stir together kefir, oats, chia seeds and vanilla. Top with blueberries.
2 Refrigerate overnight.
3 Serve with walnuts and sunflower seeds.

TIP
Meal prepping? Mix up a few pint jars of these oats (they'll keep for three days), but leave out the berries, nuts and seeds until you're ready to eat. That way, the oats will soften but the rest will stay fresh (or crunchy).

Soups, Salads & Bowls

WHO SAYS DETOX HAS TO BE A DRAG? TRY THESE YUMMY RECIPES IF YOU WANT A LIGHT LUNCH, DINNER OR MIDDAY SNACK.

Chicken Bone Broth

Bone broth is flavorful, rich and perfect to sip throughout the day. This version is easy to make in a slow cooker. Use cooked chicken bones if you've got any left from a roasted chicken. The broth will keep in the fridge for five days; freeze for longer storage.

START TO FINISH 10 minutes (plus 1 day)
SERVINGS 24

INGREDIENTS

3   pounds raw chicken bones
1   large onion, coarsely chopped
1   tablespoon apple cider vinegar
1   tablespoon minced garlic
1   tablespoon sea salt
4   fresh bay leaves
3   quarts water
GARNISH Chopped parsley

INSTRUCTIONS

1 In the pot of a slow cooker, combine bones, onion, vinegar, garlic, salt and bay leaves. Cover with water, stopping at least 1 inch from top of pot.
2 Place lid on slow cooker; cook on low for 24 hours.
3 With a slotted spoon, remove and discard solids.
4 Pour mixture through a strainer; let cool.
5 Transfer to three 1-quart glass jars with lids; store in refrigerator.
6 Garnish with parsley just before serving.

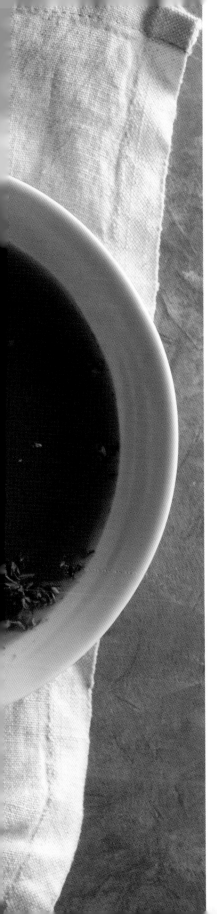

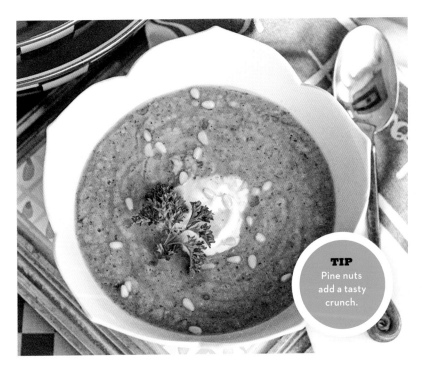

TIP
Pine nuts add a tasty crunch.

Herbed Pea & Asparagus Soup

The greens and herbs are packed with antioxidants to support the liver, kidneys and gut.

START TO FINISH 30 minutes (20 minutes active)

SERVINGS 4–6

INGREDIENTS

- 2 tablespoons grass-fed butter
- 3 cloves garlic, chopped
- 1 medium leek, sliced (about 1 cup)
- 1 medium white sweet potato, chopped (about 2–3 cups)
- ½ teaspoon sea salt
- ¼ teaspoon ground black pepper
- 3–4 cups chicken broth (or other bone broth)
- 1 cup chopped asparagus (1 inch of bottoms removed and discarded)
- 1 cup spinach
- 1 cup chopped parsley
- 1–2 tablespoons chopped mint
- 1–2 tablespoons chopped basil
- 1 cup peas (divided)

OPTIONAL GARNISHES Creme fraiche, pine nuts

INSTRUCTIONS

1 Heat butter in large pot over medium. Add garlic and leeks and saute for 1 to 2 minutes. Add sweet potato, sea salt and black pepper and saute for another 2 to 4 minutes, stirring occasionally.

2 Add broth, bring to a boil, then reduce to a simmer for about 10 to 12 minutes, until the potatoes are soft (you should be able to easily pierce them with a fork).

3 Add asparagus, spinach, parsley, mint and basil, and mix well. Continue to simmer for another 5 to 7 minutes, until greens become soft. Add ½ cup peas and mix well.

4 Blend everything with an immersion blender until smooth. Stir in remaining ½ cup peas. Garnish with creme fraiche and pine nuts, if desired.

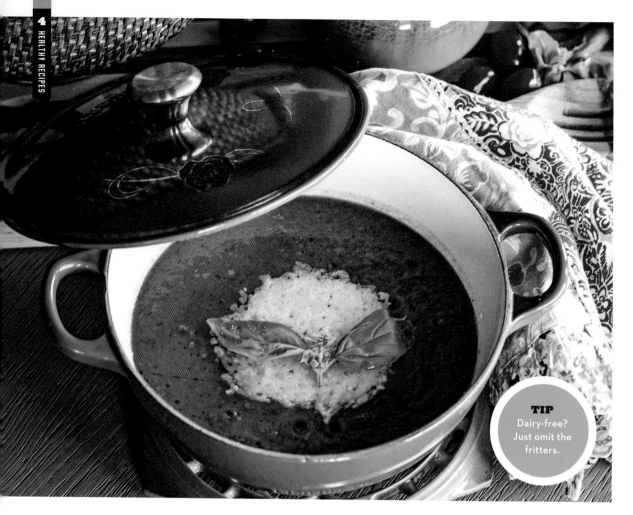

TIP
Dairy-free?
Just omit the
fritters.

Tomato Soup

Tomatoes are high in lycopene, an antioxidant that boosts the immune system. And garlic is high in vitamin C, which helps support both the immune system and liver.

START TO FINISH 1 hour (10 minutes active)
SERVINGS 4-6

INGREDIENTS

3–4 tablespoons ghee
6 cloves garlic, mashed
1 tablespoon sea salt
½ teaspoon ground black pepper
Pinch red pepper flakes
1 medium to large sweet potato, diced
3–4 cups turkey broth (or other bone broth)
2 (14.5-ounce) cans fire-roasted diced tomatoes
Parmesan Fritters (recipe below)
GARNISHES Basil, avocado oil

INSTRUCTIONS

1 In a Dutch oven, melt ghee. Add garlic, seasonings and potato, and let flavors combine for 3 to 4 minutes.
2 Add broth and tomatoes. Bring to a boil, then allow to simmer until potatoes soften (about 20 to 30 minutes).
3 Allow to cool; blend soup with an immersion blender (or in a blender in batches) until smooth and creamy. Garnish with Parmesan Fritters (see below), basil, avocado oil and sea salt.

FOR PARMESAN FRITTERS

1 Preheat oven to 400 F, and line a baking sheet with parchment paper.
2 Add a few pinches of grated Parmesan cheese, spacing each pile a couple of inches apart (like you're making cookies).
3 Bake 4 to 7 minutes to get desired level of crispiness. (Parmesan is excellent for gut health, because aging makes it higher in probiotics.)

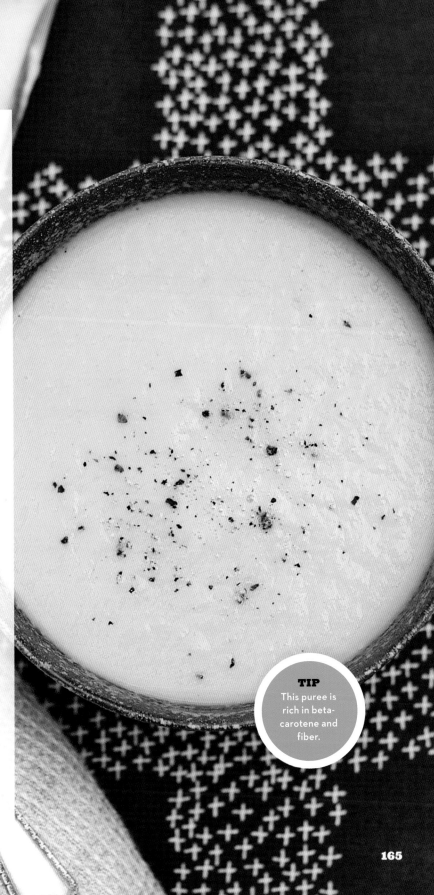

Curried Carrot Soup

Smooth, creamy and vegan to boot, this antioxidant-loaded soup works well for either lunch or dinner.

START TO FINISH 40 minutes (30 minutes active)

SERVINGS 8

INGREDIENTS

- 3 tablespoons coconut oil
- 2 teaspoons curry powder
- 8 medium carrots, peeled and thinly sliced
- 4 medium stalks celery, chopped
- 1 medium yellow onion, coarsely chopped
- 5 cups vegetable broth
- 1 tablespoon freshly squeezed lemon juice
- 2 teaspoons sea salt
- GARNISH Freshly ground black pepper to taste

INSTRUCTIONS

1 In a medium saucepan over low heat, cook coconut oil and curry powder, stirring, for 2 minutes. Stir in carrots, celery and onion, toss to coat, and cook, stirring frequently, for 10 minutes.

2 Stir in vegetable broth, bring to a boil, reduce heat to low, and simmer for 10 minutes or until vegetables are very tender. Allow to sit for 1 minute, and skim grease from top of soup if necessary.

3 In a blender, and working in batches of no more than 2 cups, puree soup. Return soup to the pot and heat through. Add lemon juice, season with sea salt and black pepper, and serve.

TIP
This puree is rich in beta-carotene and fiber.

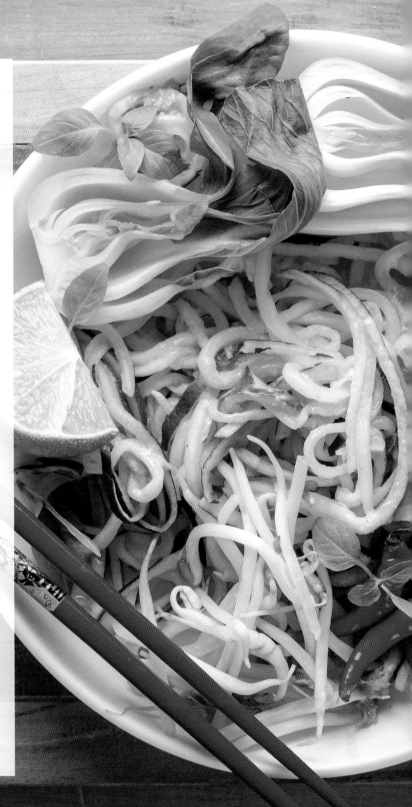

Pad Thai Zoodle Salad

Spiralized veggies lighten up this dish, while traditional seasonings keep it authentic in flavor. Zucchini promotes healthy digestion with both soluble and insoluble fiber.

START TO FINISH 15 minutes (10 minutes active)

SERVINGS 4

INGREDIENTS

- 2/3 cup peanut butter
- 6 tablespoons sesame oil, divided
- 2 tablespoons lime juice
- 1 teaspoon sea salt
- 1/2 teaspoon red pepper flakes
- 2 (7-ounce) packages zucchini zoodles
- 4 heads baby bok choy, halved lengthwise

  GARNISHES Bean sprouts, chopped peanuts, lime wedges, whole bird's-eye (Thai) chiles, Thai basil

INSTRUCTIONS

1 In a small bowl, combine peanut butter, 4 tablespoons sesame oil, lime juice, salt and red pepper flakes until smooth to make dressing. Set aside.

2 In a large skillet over medium-high heat, heat remaining sesame oil. Add zoodles and baby bok choy. Cook, stirring frequently, for 2 to 3 minutes.

3 Toss dressing with the zoodles and bok choy. Evenly divide between 4 plates.

4 Top with desired garnishes just before serving.

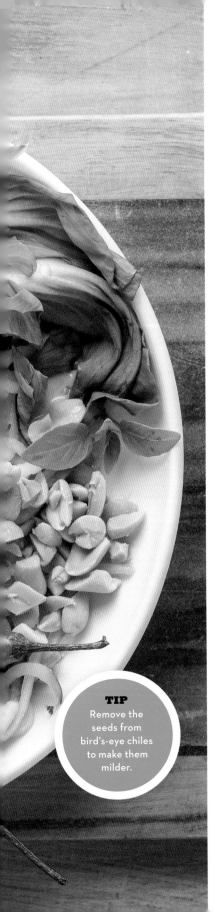

TIP
Remove the seeds from bird's-eye chiles to make them milder.

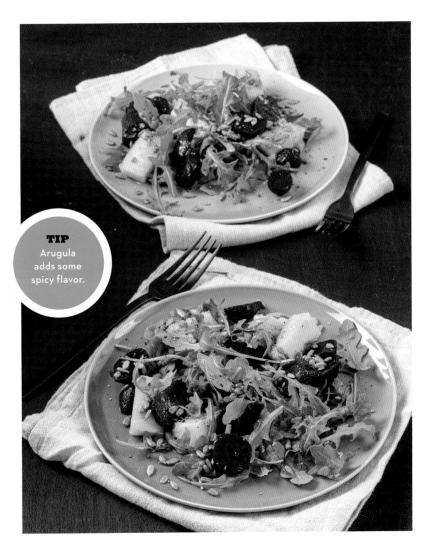

TIP
Arugula adds some spicy flavor.

Beet & Pineapple Salad With Sunflower Seeds

Pineapple contains bromelain, an enzyme that breaks down protein and aids digestion. Beets are packed with nutrients and fiber.

START TO FINISH 15 minutes (10 minutes active)

SERVINGS 4

INGREDIENTS

- 1 cup extra-virgin olive oil
- 4 tablespoons sherry vinegar
- 1 teaspoon sea salt
- ½ teaspoon ground black pepper
- 4 cups arugula
- 8 cooked beets, sliced
- 2 cups sliced fresh pineapple
- ½ cup sunflower seeds
- ½ teaspoon cracked black pepper, optional

INSTRUCTIONS

1 In a blender, combine olive oil, sherry vinegar, sea salt and pepper to make dressing.

2 Evenly divide arugula, beets, pineapple and sunflower seeds between 4 serving plates.

3 Drizzle with dressing; top with cracked black pepper, if desired.

167

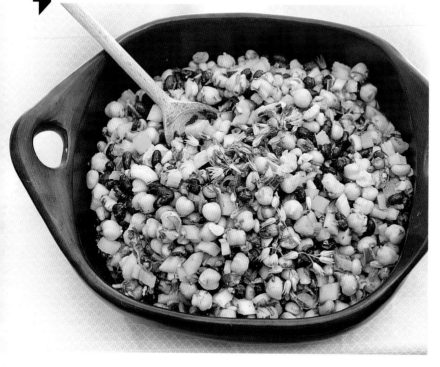

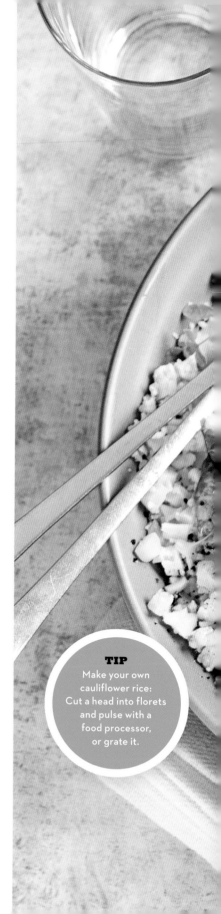

Not Your Grandma's Three-Bean Salad

A far cry from the oil-laden picnic staple of years ago, this (naturally vegan) fresh take on a classic is filled with protein, fiber and B vitamins.

START TO FINISH 20 minutes
(10 minutes active)
SERVINGS 6

INGREDIENTS

- ¼ cup olive oil
- 1 teaspoon ground cumin
- ½ teaspoon smoked paprika
- 1 (15-ounce) can black beans, drained and rinsed
- 1 (15-ounce) can black-eyed peas, drained and rinsed
- 1 (15-ounce) can chickpeas, drained and rinsed
- ½ cup chopped red onion
- 2 cups thinly sliced celery
- 2 tablespoons fresh lime juice
- 1 tablespoon apple cider vinegar
- ½ cup fresh cilantro, chopped
- 1 teaspoon finely chopped garlic
- 1½ teaspoons sea salt
- ¼ teaspoon ground black pepper

INSTRUCTIONS

1 In a small heavy skillet over moderately low heat, heat oil until hot but not smoking. Add cumin and smoked paprika, stirring until fragrant and a shade darker, about 30 seconds.

2 Pour into a large heatproof bowl. Add remaining ingredients to the cumin and smoked-paprika oil. Toss to coat. Let stand 10 minutes for flavors to blend.

TIP
Make your own cauliflower rice: Cut a head into florets and pulse with a food processor, or grate it.

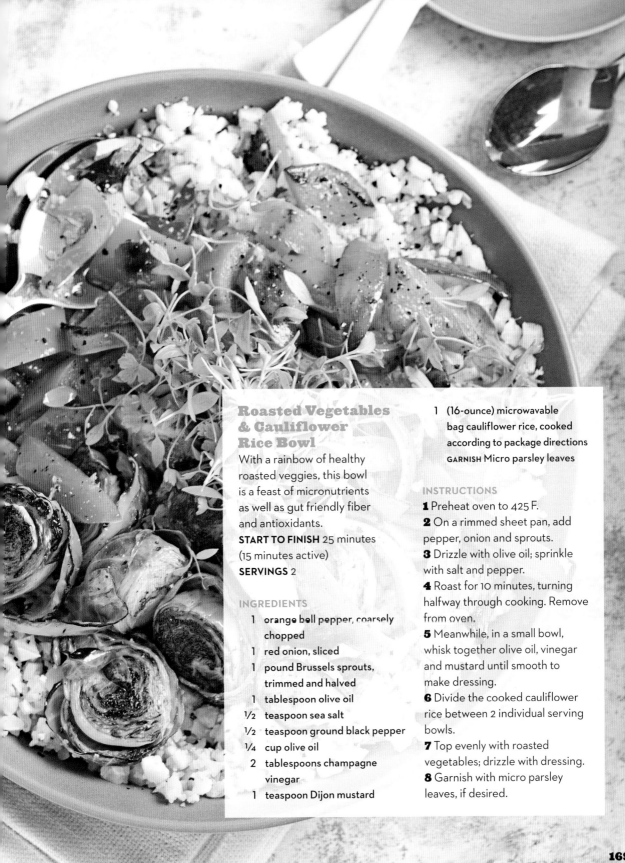

Roasted Vegetables & Cauliflower Rice Bowl

With a rainbow of healthy roasted veggies, this bowl is a feast of micronutrients as well as gut friendly fiber and antioxidants.

START TO FINISH 25 minutes (15 minutes active)
SERVINGS 2

INGREDIENTS

- 1 orange bell pepper, coarsely chopped
- 1 red onion, sliced
- 1 pound Brussels sprouts, trimmed and halved
- 1 tablespoon olive oil
- ½ teaspoon sea salt
- ½ teaspoon ground black pepper
- ¼ cup olive oil
- 2 tablespoons champagne vinegar
- 1 teaspoon Dijon mustard
- 1 (16-ounce) microwavable bag cauliflower rice, cooked according to package directions

GARNISH Micro parsley leaves

INSTRUCTIONS

1 Preheat oven to 425 F.
2 On a rimmed sheet pan, add pepper, onion and sprouts.
3 Drizzle with olive oil; sprinkle with salt and pepper.
4 Roast for 10 minutes, turning halfway through cooking. Remove from oven.
5 Meanwhile, in a small bowl, whisk together olive oil, vinegar and mustard until smooth to make dressing.
6 Divide the cooked cauliflower rice between 2 individual serving bowls.
7 Top evenly with roasted vegetables; drizzle with dressing.
8 Garnish with micro parsley leaves, if desired.

TIP
Black radish
cleanses the
liver.

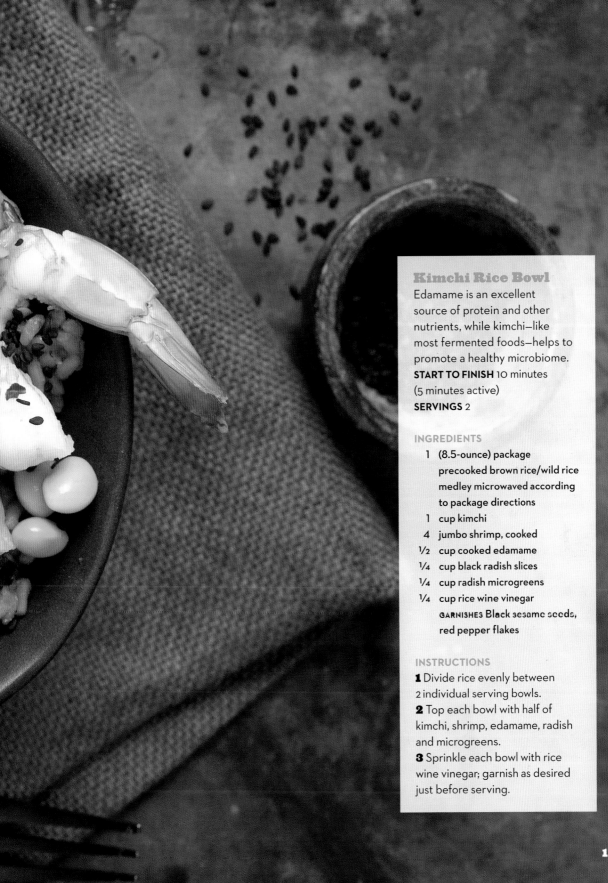

Kimchi Rice Bowl

Edamame is an excellent source of protein and other nutrients, while kimchi—like most fermented foods—helps to promote a healthy microbiome.

START TO FINISH 10 minutes (5 minutes active)
SERVINGS 2

INGREDIENTS

- 1 (8.5-ounce) package precooked brown rice/wild rice medley microwaved according to package directions
- 1 cup kimchi
- 4 jumbo shrimp, cooked
- ½ cup cooked edamame
- ¼ cup black radish slices
- ¼ cup radish microgreens
- ¼ cup rice wine vinegar
- GARNISHES Black sesame seeds, red pepper flakes

INSTRUCTIONS

1 Divide rice evenly between 2 individual serving bowls.
2 Top each bowl with half of kimchi, shrimp, edamame, radish and microgreens.
3 Sprinkle each bowl with rice wine vinegar; garnish as desired just before serving.

Main Meals

FULFILL YOUR APPETITE WITH
HEARTY RECIPES THAT STILL FIT
INTO A DETOX PROGRAM AND KEEP
YOUR CLEAN EATING ON TRACK.

Grilled Lemon Chicken & Asparagus

This simple dinner comes together quickly. Add other veggies, such as baby spinach or kale, to boost the nutrition benefits; serve with a side of brown rice.

START TO FINISH 20 minutes (10 minutes active)

SERVINGS 4

INGREDIENTS

- 4 boneless skinless chicken breasts
- ½ teaspoon salt
- ½ teaspoon ground black pepper
- 1 tablespoon avocado oil
- 1 pound asparagus, trimmed
- 2 lemons, halved
- GARNISH Parsley leaves

INSTRUCTIONS

1 Sprinkle both sides of chicken breasts with salt and pepper.

2 Brush a grill pan with avocado oil; place over medium-high heat.

3 Place chicken in pan; cook 3 to 4 minutes per side till done.

4 Set chicken aside; keep warm. In same pan, place asparagus and lemon halves (cut side down); cook for 2 minutes.

5 Divide chicken, asparagus and lemon halves among 4 dinner plates; garnish with parsley.

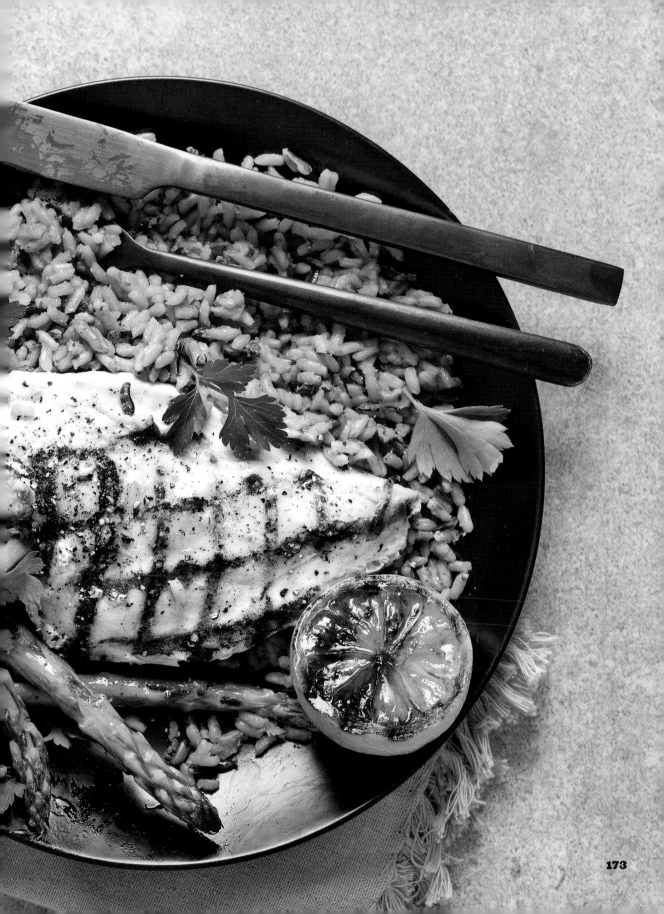

Herb-Crusted Salmon Fillets With Tomato & Oregano Salad

The herbs in this recipe give the salmon a Greek flair. Serve lemon wedges on the side; citrus and fish are a natural combo.

START TO FINISH 20 minutes (5 minutes active)

SERVINGS 4

INGREDIENTS

- 4 (6-ounce) salmon fillets
- ½ teaspoon salt
- ½ teaspoon ground black pepper
- 1 tablespoon chopped chives
- 1 tablespoon fresh dill
- 1 tablespoon fresh thyme
- 2 tablespoons avocado oil
- 1 pint cherry tomatoes, halved
- ¼ cup olive oil
- 2 cups mixed salad greens

  GARNISHES Oregano leaves, dill sprigs

INSTRUCTIONS

1 Sprinkle salmon fillets with salt, pepper and herbs.

2 In a cast-iron skillet over medium-high heat, heat avocado oil. Add fillets to pan and cook 3 minutes per side or until cooked through.

3 Meanwhile, in a large bowl, toss tomato halves with olive oil.

4 Divide salad greens among 4 dinner plates.

5 Top the greens with salmon and tomatoes. Garnish with oregano leaves and dill.

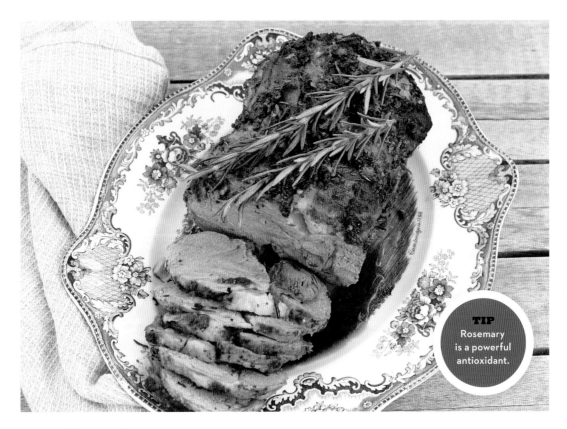

TIP
Rosemary is a powerful antioxidant.

Herb-Crusted Lamb Roast

Lamb is nutrient dense, and a great source of protein, healthy fats and iron. It's also rich in B vitamins such as B12 and B6, which promote a healthy nervous system, and zinc, which supports a healthy immune response. Plus, you'll have lots of leftovers for salads and snacks!

START TO FINISH About 3 hours (10 minutes active)

SERVINGS 8–10

INGREDIENTS

- 8 cloves garlic, peeled
- ¼ cup fresh mint
- 1 small bunch flat-leaf parsley
- 4 tablespoons fresh rosemary
- 2 tablespoons lemon zest
- 1 teaspoon sea salt, plus more for seasoning
- 1 teaspoon ground black pepper, plus more for seasoning
- ¼ cup olive oil
- 1 (4–5 pound) boneless lamb roast, tied up with string
- GARNISH Rosemary sprigs

INSTRUCTIONS

1 In a food processor fitted with the S blade, add garlic, mint, parsley, rosemary, lemon zest, sea salt, pepper and oil. Process until finely chopped.

2 Season the lamb with a small amount of salt and pepper on all sides. Coat the top and sides of the lamb with the herb mixture. Allow to sit at room temperature for 30 minutes to 1 hour.

3 While lamb is resting, preheat oven to 450 F. Set the oven rack in the lower third of the oven so the lamb will sit in the middle of the oven. Place lamb in a large roasting pan. Roast for 1¼ to 1½ hours, or until the internal temperature of the lamb reaches 135 F (for rare) or 145 F (for medium).

4 Remove lamb from the oven and place on a platter; cover tightly with foil and let rest for about 20 minutes before slicing. Garnish with rosemary sprigs.

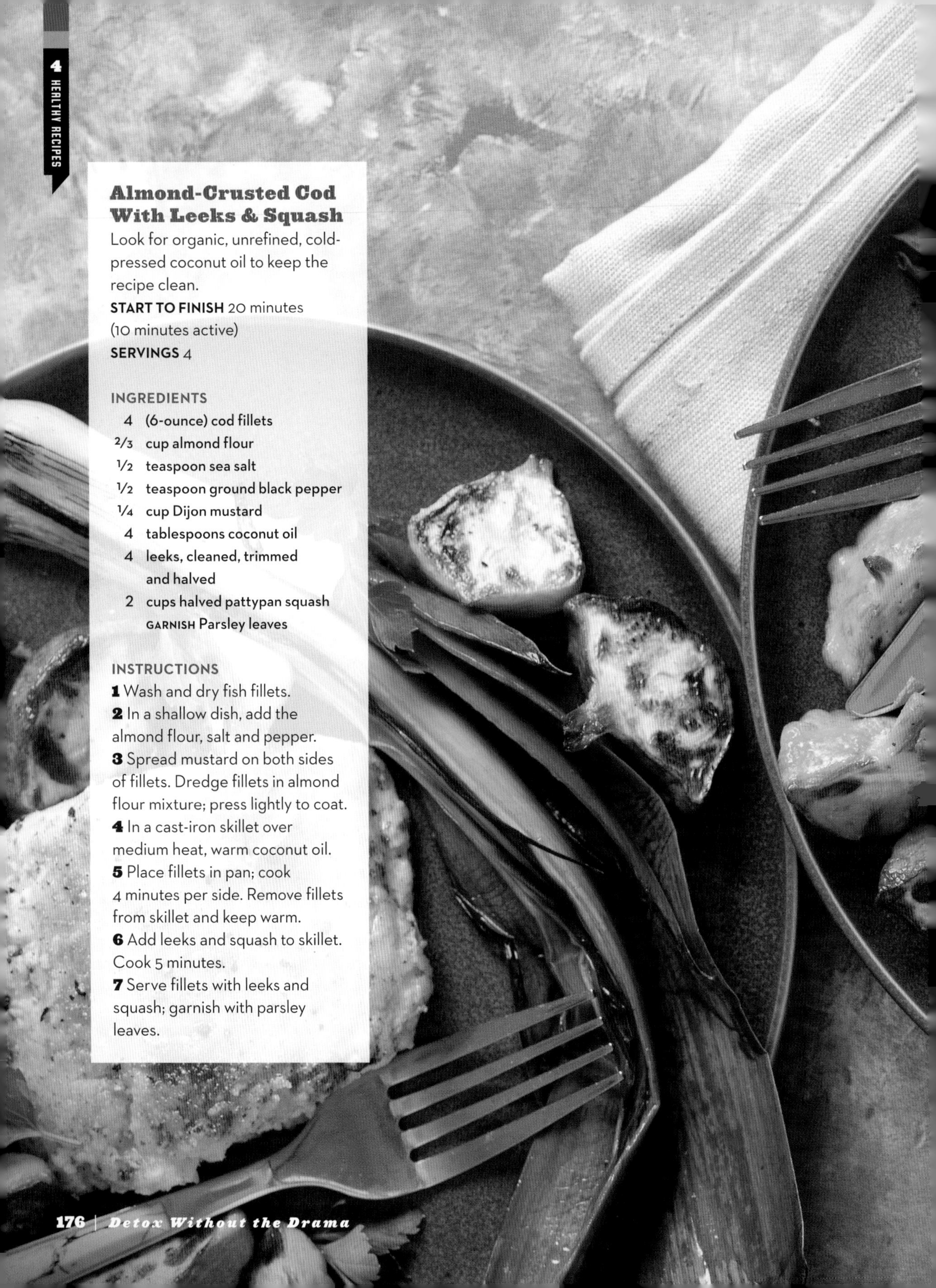

Almond-Crusted Cod With Leeks & Squash

Look for organic, unrefined, cold-pressed coconut oil to keep the recipe clean.

START TO FINISH 20 minutes (10 minutes active)

SERVINGS 4

INGREDIENTS

- 4   (6-ounce) cod fillets
- 2/3   cup almond flour
- 1/2   teaspoon sea salt
- 1/2   teaspoon ground black pepper
- 1/4   cup Dijon mustard
- 4   tablespoons coconut oil
- 4   leeks, cleaned, trimmed and halved
- 2   cups halved pattypan squash

GARNISH Parsley leaves

INSTRUCTIONS

1 Wash and dry fish fillets.
2 In a shallow dish, add the almond flour, salt and pepper.
3 Spread mustard on both sides of fillets. Dredge fillets in almond flour mixture; press lightly to coat.
4 In a cast-iron skillet over medium heat, warm coconut oil.
5 Place fillets in pan; cook 4 minutes per side. Remove fillets from skillet and keep warm.
6 Add leeks and squash to skillet. Cook 5 minutes.
7 Serve fillets with leeks and squash; garnish with parsley leaves.

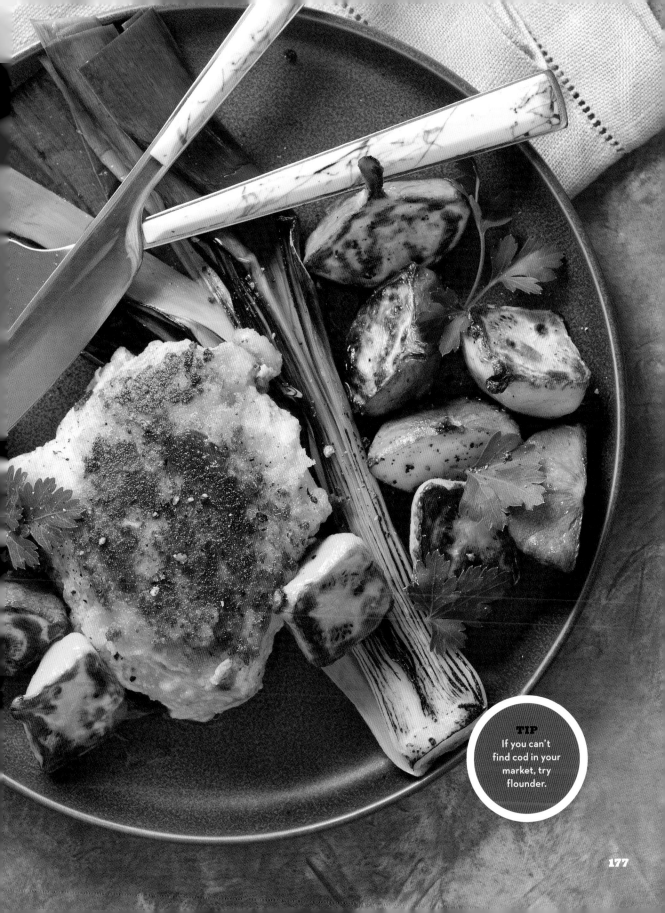

TIP
If you can't find cod in your market, try flounder.

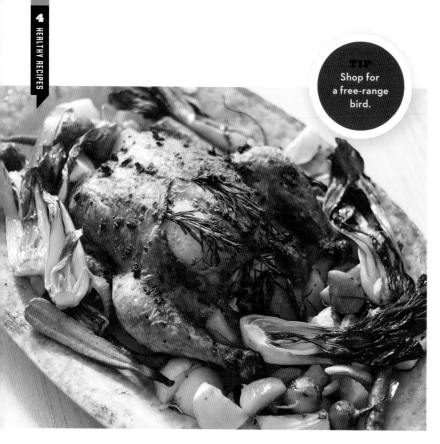

TIP
Shop for
a free-range
bird.

Garlic-Roasted Chicken With Vegetables

The antioxidant-packed medley of vegetables cooks along with the chicken—rubbed with turmeric, a potent anti-inflammatory spice—to make a complete dinner. Then you'll have leftovers for salads and lettuce wraps.

START TO FINISH 2 hours (10 minutes active)

SERVINGS 4

INGREDIENTS

FOR THE CHICKEN

- 1 (5–6 pound) organic roasting chicken
- 8 cloves garlic, minced finely
- 1 lemon, quartered
- 2 sprigs fresh rosemary
- 1½ teaspoons sea salt
- 1 teaspoon freshly ground black pepper
- 1 teaspoon turmeric
- 2 tablespoons olive oil

FOR THE VEGETABLES

- 1 bulb fennel, sliced and fronds removed (you can stuff fronds into the bird's cavity)
- 1 bunch radishes, stems trimmed
- 3 golden beets, peeled and quartered
- 3 small yellow onions, peeled and quartered
- 5 carrots, halved
- 2 turnips, peeled and quartered
- 3 small heads bok choy, halved
- 3 cloves garlic, smashed
- 1 tablespoon olive oil
- 2 sprigs fresh rosemary
  Sea salt and freshly ground black pepper to taste

INSTRUCTIONS

1 Preheat oven to 425 F. Remove the bag of chicken giblets. Rinse the chicken inside and out, and pat dry with a paper towel. Loosen the skin on the breast of the chicken and rub the garlic under the skin and on the meat.

2 Stuff the bird's cavity with the lemon and rosemary. In a small bowl, combine the salt, pepper and turmeric. Rub the outside of the chicken with the spice mixture. Place the chicken in a roasting pan; tuck the wing tips under the body of the chicken so they don't burn. Drizzle the chicken with olive oil.

3 Roast the chicken for 1½ hours, or until the juices run clear when you cut between a leg and thigh (or to an internal temperature of 165 F).

4 Meanwhile, about halfway through cooking, prepare the vegetables: Toss all ingredients together, season with salt and pepper, and spread on a parchment-lined baking sheet. Cook for 45 minutes, turning vegetables occasionally until they get a little caramelized.

5 When chicken reaches the proper internal temperature, remove it from the oven, place it on a serving platter, and cover with foil; let rest for about 20 minutes.

6 While chicken rests, remove vegetables from oven; discard rosemary stems.

7 Arrange the vegetables around the chicken and serve (slice the chicken just before serving).

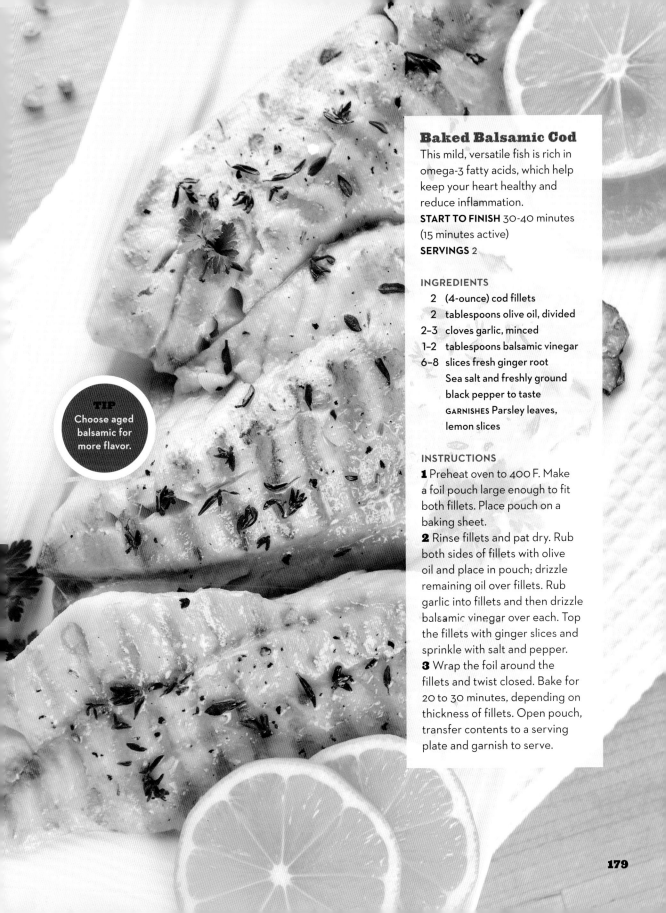

Baked Balsamic Cod

This mild, versatile fish is rich in omega-3 fatty acids, which help keep your heart healthy and reduce inflammation.

START TO FINISH 30-40 minutes (15 minutes active)

SERVINGS 2

INGREDIENTS

 2 (4-ounce) cod fillets
 2 tablespoons olive oil, divided
2-3 cloves garlic, minced
1-2 tablespoons balsamic vinegar
6-8 slices fresh ginger root
     Sea salt and freshly ground black pepper to taste
     GARNISHES Parsley leaves, lemon slices

INSTRUCTIONS

1 Preheat oven to 400 F. Make a foil pouch large enough to fit both fillets. Place pouch on a baking sheet.

2 Rinse fillets and pat dry. Rub both sides of fillets with olive oil and place in pouch; drizzle remaining oil over fillets. Rub garlic into fillets and then drizzle balsamic vinegar over each. Top the fillets with ginger slices and sprinkle with salt and pepper.

3 Wrap the foil around the fillets and twist closed. Bake for 20 to 30 minutes, depending on thickness of fillets. Open pouch, transfer contents to a serving plate and garnish to serve.

TIP Choose aged balsamic for more flavor.

179

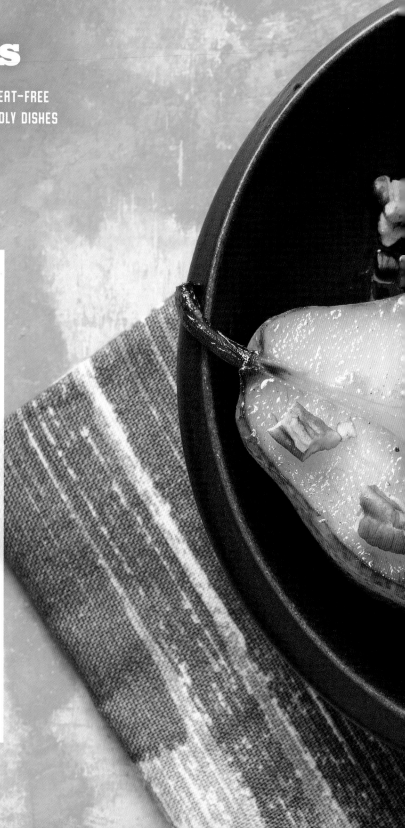

Desserts

DETOX DOESN'T HAVE TO BE A TREAT-FREE ZONE. TRY THESE CLEANSE-FRIENDLY DISHES TO SATISFY YOUR SWEET TOOTH.

Baked Pears With Pecans

These pears are yummy on their own, or top them with whipped coconut cream or dairy-free ice cream.

START TO FINISH 30 minutes (5 minutes active)

SERVINGS 4

INGREDIENTS

- 4 tablespoons dark brown sugar
- 2 tablespoons coconut oil
- ½ cup water
- ¼ teaspoon nutmeg
- 4 Bosc pears, halved and cored
- 4 tablespoons chopped pecans

INSTRUCTIONS

1 Preheat oven to 350 F.

2 In a small bowl, combine dark brown sugar, coconut oil, water and nutmeg.

3 Place cored pear halves in an ovenproof dish; pour brown sugar mixture over pears; bake for 25 minutes or until soft and tender.

4 Sprinkle with chopped pecans; serve warm.

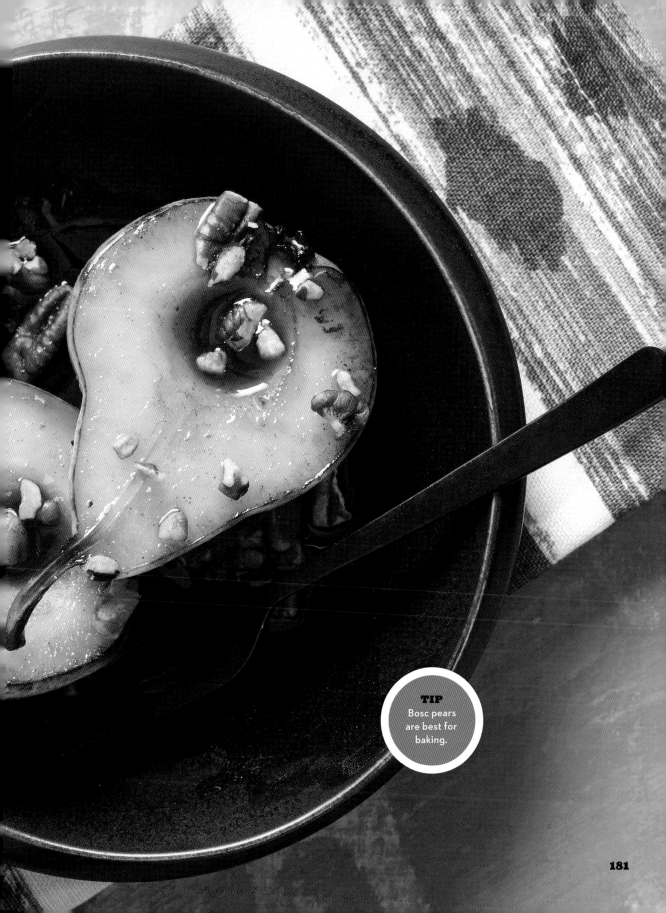

TIP
Bosc pears are best for baking.

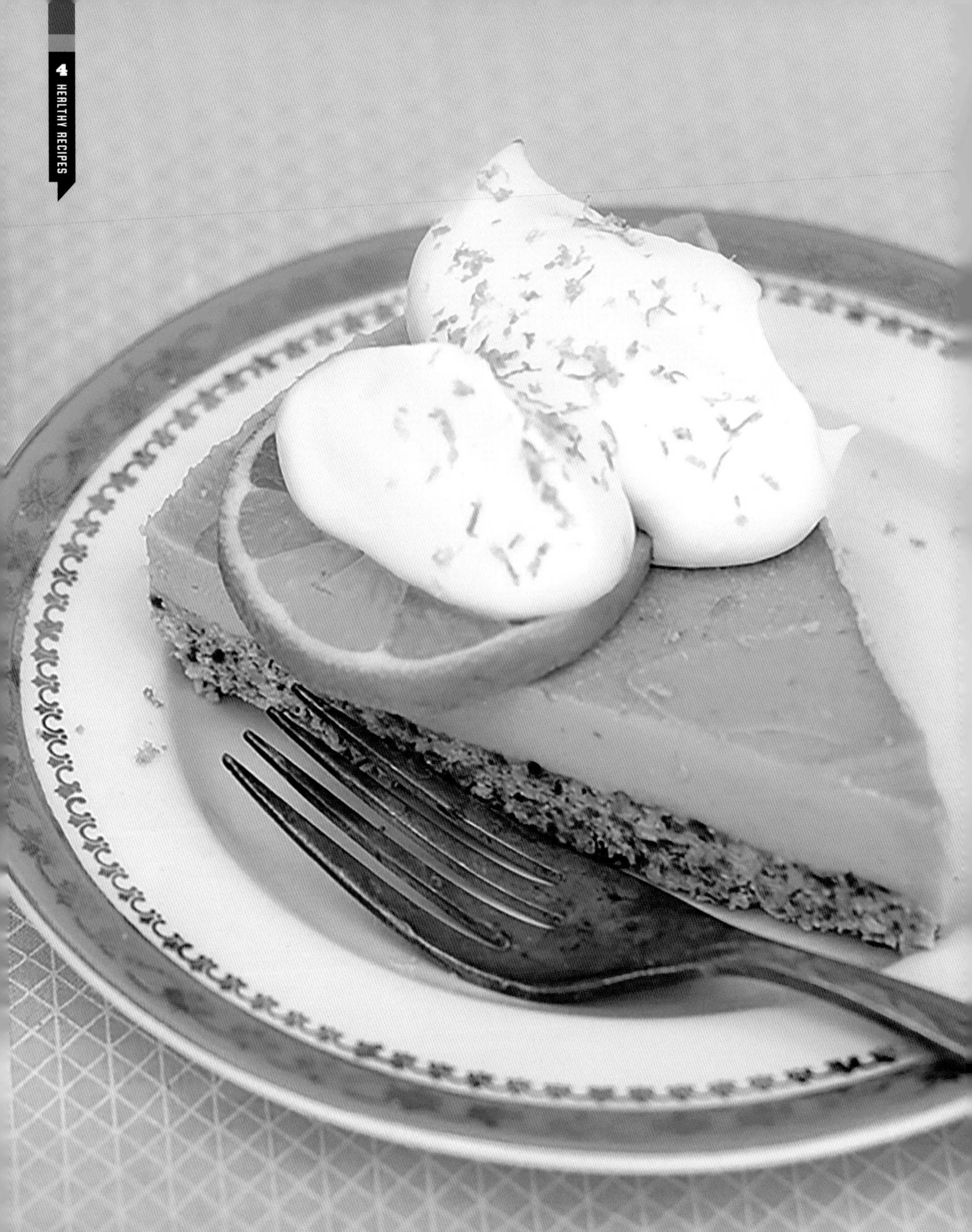

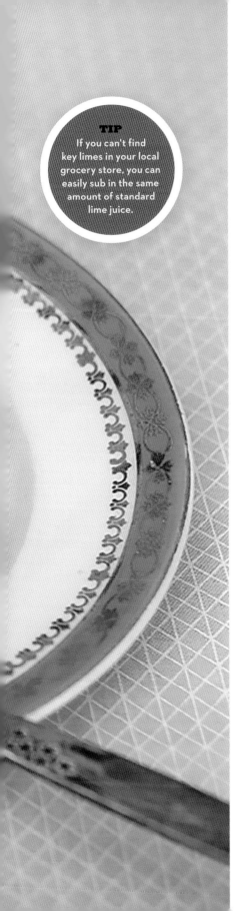

Raw Key Lime & Vanilla Bean Tart

Free from gluten and dairy, two major allergens, this flavorful, naturally sweet tart sidesteps the usual crash-and-burn you get from sugary treats.

START TO FINISH 4 to 12 hours (15 minutes active)

SERVINGS 10

INGREDIENTS

FOR THE CRUST

- 2 cups raw, unsalted cashews
- ½ cup shredded, unsweetened coconut
- 1 cup dates, pitted
- ⅛ teaspoon sea salt

FOR THE FILLING

- 1 large avocado, pitted and peeled
- 1 cup raw cashews, soaked in water for at least 2 hours and drained
- ½ cup melted coconut oil
- ¼ cup freshly squeezed lime juice
- ½ cup maple syrup
- 1 vanilla bean, scraped
  Pinch sea salt
- 1 tablespoon lime zest
  Coconut Whipped Cream (recipe follows)

INSTRUCTIONS

1 To make the crust: In a food processor fitted with an S blade, add all crust ingredients. Process until the ingredients are mixed and finely broken down, sticking together when you squeeze a small handful. Press crust ingredients into the bottom of an oiled 9-inch springform pan.

2 To make the filling: Using a high-speed blender, blend together all filling ingredients until smooth. Spread the filling over the crust, using a spatula to make the top very smooth.

3 Chill the pie in the freezer for an hour, then transfer it to the fridge and let it set for another 3 hours, or overnight. Cut into slices and serve with Coconut Whipped Cream.

FOR COCONUT WHIPPED CREAM

- 13.5 ounces full-fat canned organic coconut milk, refrigerated overnight
- 1½ tablespoons honey
- 1½ teaspoons vanilla extract

INSTRUCTIONS

1 Carefully open the can of refrigerated coconut milk. Keeping can level, scrape out thick, waxy top layer of coconut cream and place in a mixing bowl. (Save leftover coconut water from can for a shake or smoothie.)

2 Using a hand or stand mixer on high speed, whip the coconut cream for 3 minutes until it becomes light and fluffy. Add honey and vanilla and whip for 2 more minutes.

183

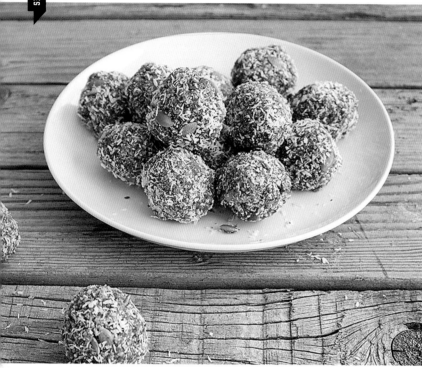

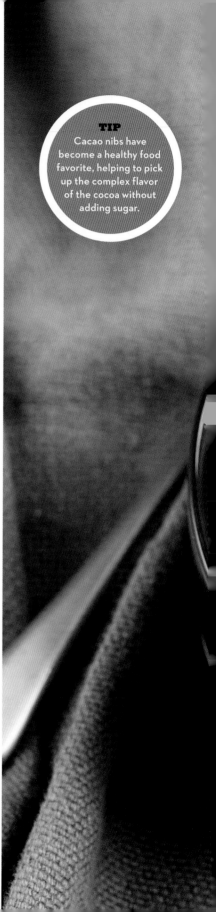

TIP
Cacao nibs have become a healthy food favorite, helping to pick up the complex flavor of the cocoa without adding sugar.

Nut-Free Joy Balls

Enjoy these nut-free treats as a grab-and-go dessert. This recipe features nutrient-packed seeds, including flaxseeds, which are rich in omega-3 fatty acids.

START TO FINISH About 2 hours (15 minutes active)
SERVINGS Yields 3 dozen

INGREDIENTS

  1   cup raw sunflower seeds
  1   cup raw pumpkin seeds, divided
 ¼   cup ground flaxseed
  1   teaspoon cinnamon
      Pinch of sea salt
  1   cup dried dates, pitted
  2   tablespoons maple syrup
 ½   cup raisins
 ½   cup unsweetened shredded
      dried coconut (optional)

INSTRUCTIONS

1 In a food processor fitted with an S blade, combine sunflower seeds, ½ cup pumpkin seeds, ground flaxseed, cinnamon and sea salt, and process for 1 to 2 minutes until fine. Add dates and maple syrup, and process again until a thick paste forms. Mixture will be sticky and dense.

2 Transfer to a bowl and, using your hands, mix in the remaining ½ cup pumpkin seeds and the raisins. Roll small amounts of the mixture between your palms to form 1-inch balls. Roll balls in shredded coconut to coat (optional).

3 Place in a container with a tight-fitting lid and refrigerate or freeze. Serve chilled or frozen.

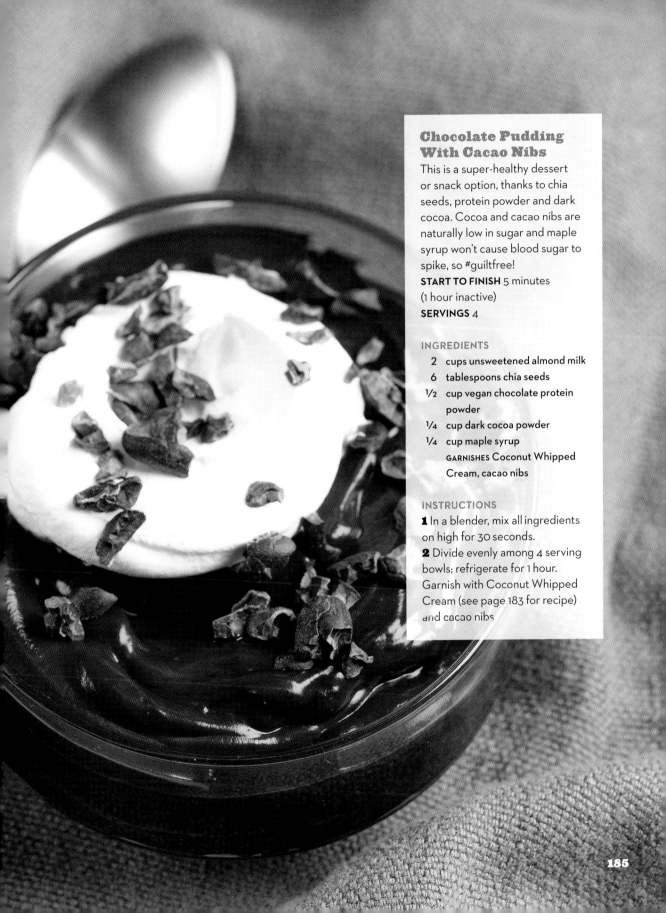

Chocolate Pudding With Cacao Nibs

This is a super-healthy dessert or snack option, thanks to chia seeds, protein powder and dark cocoa. Cocoa and cacao nibs are naturally low in sugar and maple syrup won't cause blood sugar to spike, so #guiltfree!

START TO FINISH 5 minutes (1 hour inactive)
SERVINGS 4

INGREDIENTS

- 2 cups unsweetened almond milk
- 6 tablespoons chia seeds
- ½ cup vegan chocolate protein powder
- ¼ cup dark cocoa powder
- ¼ cup maple syrup
- GARNISHES Coconut Whipped Cream, cacao nibs

INSTRUCTIONS

1 In a blender, mix all ingredients on high for 30 seconds.
2 Divide evenly among 4 serving bowls; refrigerate for 1 hour. Garnish with Coconut Whipped Cream (see page 183 for recipe) and cacao nibs.

CREDITS

COVER fortyforks/iStockphoto/Getty Images FRONT FLAP *From top:* nensuria/iStockphoto/Getty Images; LdF/Getty Images 2-3 nensuria/iStockphoto/Getty Images 4-5 *Clockwise from top left:* Deagreez/iStockphoto/Getty Images; Claudia Totir/Getty Images; BONNINSTUDIO/Stocksy; Robert Daly/OJO Images RF/Getty Images; Photography by Liam Franklin, Recipe Styling and Development by Margaret Monroe; ma-k/Getty Images; PeopleImages/E+/Getty Images 6-7 Satyrenko/iStockphoto/Getty Images 8-9 Maria Fuchs/Cultura RF/Getty Images 10-11 *From left:* fortyforks/iStockphoto/Getty Images; PeopleImages/E+/Getty Images 12-13 Fuzullhanum/iStockphoto/Getty Images 14-15 *From left:* Dragan Grkic/EyeEm/Getty Images; LdF/Getty Images 16-17 Claudia Totir/Getty Images 18-19 PeopleImages/E+/Getty Images 20-21 LightFieldStudios/iStockphoto/Getty Images 22-23 Heritage Images/Getty Images 24-25 Ghislain & Marie David de Lossy/Cultura RF/Getty Images 26-27 cyano66/iStockphoto/Getty Images 28-29 *From left:* mikroman6/Moment RF/Getty Images; Chris Clor/Tetra images RF/Getty Images 30-31 Dkart/iStockphoto/Getty Images 32-33 Pornpak Khunatorn/iStockphoto/Getty Images 34-35 *From left:* Dkart/iStockphoto/Getty Images; SHUBHANGI GANESHRAO KENE/Science Photo Library/Getty Images 36-37 Amy Sussman/SHJ2019/Getty Images 38-39 *Clockwise from top left:* Astrid Stawiarz/Getty Images; Jeff Kravitz/Getty Images; Dimitrios Kambouris/Getty Images; Leon Bennett/Stringer/Getty Images; Kevin Winter/Getty Images; Presley Ann/Stringer/Getty Images 40-41 Courtesy Resorts (3) 42-43 yoh4nnE+/Getty Images 44-45 swissmediavision/E+/Getty Images 46-47 Agnieszka Marcinska/EyeEm/Getty Images 48-49 Westend61/Getty Images 50-51 *From left:* Lesia_G/Lesya Gapchuk/Getty Images; KatarzynaBialasiewicz/iStockphoto/Getty Images 52-53 *From left:* asbe/iStockphoto/Getty Images; 2Mmedia/iStockphoto/Getty Images 54-55 draganab/E+/Getty Images 56-57 Lena Clara/Getty Images 58-59 Deagreez/iStockphoto/Getty Images 60-61 andresr/Getty Images 62-63 *From left:* Oleksii Polishchuk/iStockphoto/Getty Images; Antagain/E+/Getty Images 64-65 golfcphoto/iStockphoto/Getty Images 66-67 vitapix/Getty Images 68-69 vm/E+/Getty Images 70-71 filadendron/E+/Getty Images 72-73 PeopleImages/E+/Getty Images 74-75 *From left:* chee gin tan/E+/Getty Images; dusanpetkovic/iStockphoto/Getty Images 76-77 *From left:* uniquely india/Getty Images; Michael Rowe/Digital Vision/Getty Images; fizkes/iStockphoto/Getty Images 78-79 SrdjanPav/Getty Images 80-81 JGI/Jamie Grill/Tetra images RF/Getty Images 82-83 Olga Strogonova/EyeEm/Getty Images 84-85 *From left:* moodboard/Cultura RF/Getty Images 86-87 Ingo Rösler/Getty Images 88-89 *From left:* PeopleImages/Getty Images; Farknot Architect/Alamy Stock Photo 90-91 *From left:* GlobalStock/iStockphoto; Colin Anderson Productions pty l/Getty Images 92-93 *Clockwise from left:* Alex Brunsdon/Getty Images; Science Photo Library RF/Getty Images; Creativ Studio Heinemann/Getty Images; Robert Daly/OJO Images RF/Getty Images; Creativ Studio Heinemann/Getty Images; EivaislaiStockphoto/Getty Images; Brian Hagiwara/Getty Images 94-95 *From left:* Dimitris66/E+/Getty Images; Jenny Dettrick/Getty Images; StockFood/Foodcollection/Getty Images; Juno/Stocksy 96-97 *From left:* Darren Muir/Stocksy; ZenShui/Michele Constantini/PhotoAlto/Getty Images; ROTTSTRA/E+/Getty Images 98-99 *From left:* Alita Ong/Stocksy; Lew Robertson/Getty Images; Natasha_Avdeyuk/Screen moment/Stocksy 100-101 *Clockwise from top left:* Coprid/iStockphoto/Getty Images; Floortje/iStockphoto/Getty Images; Brian Hagiwara/Getty Images; Giulia Cosci/iStockphoto/Getty Images; hdere/E+/Getty Images; Image Source/Getty Images; Creative-Family/iStockphoto/Getty Images; taffpix/iStockphoto/Getty Images; Rosemary Calvert/Getty Images; Sezeryadigar/E+/Getty Images; colnihko/iStockphoto/Getty Images; Magone/iStockphoto/Getty Images; Annabelle Breakey/Stockbyte/Getty Images; Aniko Hobel/Moment RF/Getty Images 102-103 andresr/E+/Getty Images 104-105 apichon_tee/iStockphoto/Getty Images 106-107 *From left:* fcafotodigital/iStockphoto/Getty Images; Jose Luis Pelaez Inc/Getty Images 108-109 Daniel Kim Photography/Stocksy 110-111 *From left:* Svetl/iStockphoto/Getty Images; Westend61/Getty Images 112-113 Daly and Newton/OJO Images RF/Getty Images 114-115 MIA Studio/Shutterstock 116-117 *From left:* BONNINSTUDIO/Stocksy; StockFood/Foodcollection/Getty Images 118-119 gilaxia/Getty Images 120-121 Prostock-Studio/iStockphoto/Getty Images 122-123 Dimitri Otis/Getty Images 124-125 Yulia Reznikov/Getty Images 126-127 Larry Washburn/fStop/Getty Images 128-129 *From left:* Robert Daly/Getty Images; Jordan Lutes/Image Source/Getty Images 130-131 Foxys_forest_manufacture/iStockphoto/Getty Images 132-133 photomaru/iStockphoto/Getty Images 134-135 Courtesy of Jo Schaalman and Jules Peláez of The Conscious Cleanse 136-137 Image Source/Getty Images 138-139 *From left:* Science Photo Library/Getty Images; ma-k/Getty Images 140-141 MARC TRAN/Stocksy 142-143 Mint Images RF/Getty Images 144-145 Hero Images/Getty Images 146-147 mimage photography/Shutterstock 148-149 Povozniuk/iStockphoto/Getty Images 150, 158, 163-165, 168, 175, 178-179, 182-184 Courtesy of Jo Schaalman and Jules Peláez of The Conscious Cleanse (11) 151-155 JACQUELINE STOFSICK (5) 156-157, 159-162, 166-167, 169-174, 176-177, 180-181, 185 Photography by Liam Franklin, Recipe Styling and Development by Margaret Monroe (14) BACK FLAP *Clockwise from top:* fortyforks/iStockphoto/Getty Images; Jenny Dettrick/Getty Images; Creativ Studio Heinemann/Westend61/Getty Images (2); ROTTSTRA/Getty Images BACK COVER *Clockwise from top left:* Robert Daly/OJO Images RF/Getty Images; Prostock-Studio/iStockphoto/Getty Images; vm/E+/Getty Images; Satyrenko/iStockphoto/Getty Images

Special Thanks to Contributing Writers

Claire Connors, Margaret Monroe, Jules Peláez, Phillip Rhodes, Jo Schaalman, Carley Smith

CENTENNIAL BOOKS

An Imprint of
Centennial Media, LLC
1111 Brickell Avenue, 10th Floor
Miami, FL 33131, U.S.A.

CENTENNIAL BOOKS is a trademark of Centennial Media, LLC

ISBN 978-1-951274-94-8

Distributed by
Simon & Schuster, Inc.
1230 Avenue of the Americas
New York, NY 10020, U.S.A.

For information about custom editions, special sales and premium and corporate purchases, please contact Centennial Media at contact@centennialmedia.com.

Manufactured in China

10 9 8 7 6 5 4 3 2 1

PUBLISHERS & CO-FOUNDERS Ben Harris, Sebastian Raatz
EDITORIAL DIRECTOR Annabel Vered
CREATIVE DIRECTOR Jessica Power
EXECUTIVE EDITOR Janet Giovanelli
FEATURES EDITOR Alyssa Shaffer
DEPUTY EDITORS Ron Kelly, Anne Marie O'Connor
MANAGING EDITOR Lisa Chambers
DESIGN DIRECTOR Martin Elfers
SENIOR ART DIRECTOR Pino Impastato
ART DIRECTORS Runyon Hall, Jaclyn Loney, Natali Suasnavas, Joseph Ulatowski
COPY/PRODUCTION Patty Carroll, Angela Taormina
SENIOR PHOTO EDITOR Jenny Veiga
PHOTO EDITOR Kim Kuhn
PRODUCTION MANAGER Paul Rodina
PRODUCTION ASSISTANT Alyssa Swiderski
EDITORIAL ASSISTANT Tiana Schippa
SALES & MARKETING Jeremy Nurnberg